Social Theory, Social Change and Social Work

Social work is currently experiencing an important period of change in its priorities, organisation and day-to-day practices. In the light of recent legislation in community care, child care and criminal justice together with changes in local government and education and training, the nature and future of social work is changing dramatically. Increasingly, notions of care management, monitoring and evaluation and inter-agency coordination become more dominant, requiring new skills and new forms of knowledge to the extent that the image of the generic social worker working in the unified agency and drawing upon casework, informed by particular forms of psychology and displaying particular skills in human relationships, seems outmoded.

Social Theory, Social Change and Social Work has two inter-related themes. First, to account for and analyse current changes in social work, and second, to assess how far recent developments in social theory can contribute to their interpretation. The book locates social work in its social and political contexts, paying particular attention to the changing organization of social work; the questions of feminism and difference; social workers as surface performers; the centrality and significance of risk; the past and futures of social work in probation, with older people and in child welfare; and social-work education and the role of CCETSW.

It will be essential reading for students on qualifying and post-qualifying social work programmes, as well as courses in sociology, social policy, politics, law and health.

Nigel Parton is Professor in Child Care at the University of Huddersfield.

The State of Welfare
Edited by Mary Langan

Nearly half a century after its post-war consolidation, the British welfare state is once again at the centre of political controversy. After a decade in which the role of the state in the provision of welfare was steadily reduced in favour of the private, voluntary and informal sectors, with relatively little public debate or resistance, the further extension of the new mixed economy of welfare in the spheres of health and education became a major political issue in the early 1990s. At the same time the impact of deepening recession has begun to expose some of the deficiencies of market forces in areas, such as housing and income maintenance, where their role had expanded dramatically during the 1980s. *The State of Welfare* provides a forum for continuing the debate about the services we need in the 1990s.

Social Theory, Social Change and Social Work

Edited by Nigel Parton

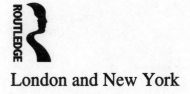

London and New York

First published 1996
by Routledge
11 New Fetter Lane, London EC4P 4EE

Simultaneously published in the USA and Canada
by Routledge
29 West 35th Street, New York, NY 10001

Reprinted in 1996

© 1996 Nigel Parton, selection and editorial matter;
individual chapters, the contributors

Typeset in Times by
Ponting–Green Publishing Services, Chesham, Bucks
Printed and bound in Great Britain by
Mackays of Chatham PLC, Chatham, Kent

British Library Cataloguing in Publication Data
A catalogue record for this book is available from the
British Library

Library of Congress Cataloguing in Publication Data
Social theory, social change and social work / edited by Nigel
Parton.
        p. cm. – (State of welfare)
    Includes bibliographical references and index.
        ISBN 0–415–12697–5 (alk. paper). –
ISBN 0–415–12698–3 (pbk : alk. paper)
1. Social service–Great Britain.
2. Social service–Great Britain–Methodology.
3. Social change–Great Britain.
4. Public welfare administration–Great Britain.
I. Parton, Nigel.   II. Series.
HV248.S634   1996
361.941–dc20   95–31962
                                                    CIP

ISBN   0–415–12697–5 (hbk)
ISBN   0–415–12698–3 (pbk)

Contents

Series editor's preface

In the 1990s the perception of a crisis of welfare systems has become universal across the Western world. The coincidence of global economic slump and the ending of the Cold War has intensified pressures to reduce welfare spending at the same time that Western governments, traditional social institutions and political parties all face unprecedented problems of legitimacy. Given the importance of welfare policies in securing popular consent for existing regimes and in maintaining social stability, welfare budgets have in general proved remarkably resilient even in the face of governments proclaiming the principles of austerity and self-reliance.

Yet the crisis of welfare has led to measures of reform and retrenchment which have provoked often bitter controversy in virtually every sphere, from hospitals and schools to social security benefits and personal social services. What is striking is the crumbling of the old structures and policies before any clear alternative has emerged. The general impression is one of exhaustion and confusion. There is a widespread sense that everything has been tried and has failed and that nobody is very clear about how to advance into an increasingly bleak future.

On both sides of the Atlantic, the agenda of free market anti-statism has provided the cutting edge for measures of privatisation. The result has been a substantial shift in the 'mixed economy' of welfare towards a more market-orientated approach. But it has not taken long for the defects of the market as a mechanism for social regulation to become apparent. Yet now that the inadequacy of the market in providing equitable or even efficient welfare services is exposed, where else is there to turn?

The *State of Welfare* series aims to provide a critical assessment of the policy implications of some of the wide social and economic changes of the 1990s. Globalisation, the emergence of post-industrial society, the transformation of work, demographic shifts and changes in gender roles and family structures all have major consequences for the patterns of welfare provision established half a century ago.

The demands of women and minority ethnic groups, as well as the voices of younger, older and disabled people and the influence of social movements concerned with issues of sexuality, gender and the environment must all be taken into account in the construction of a social policy for the new millennium.

Mary Langan
March 1995

Contributors

John Clarke Senior Lecturer in Social Policy, Faculty of Social Sciences The Open University, England.

Robert Harris Professor of Social Work and Pro Vice-Chancellor, University of Hull, England.

Jeff Hopkins, Lecturer in Social Work, Department of Applied Social Studies, University of Keele, England.

David Howe Professor of Social Work, School of Social Work, University of East Anglia, England.

Chris Jones Professor of Social Work and Social Policy, Department of Sociology, Social Policy and Social Work, University of Liverpool, England.

Olive Otway Lecturer in Social Work, Department of Applied Social Studies, University of Keele, England.

Nigel Parton Professor in Child Care, School of Human and Health Sciences, University of Huddersfield, England.

Judith Phillips Lecturer in Social Work, Department of Applied Social Studies, University of Keele, England.

David Webb Professor of Social Sciences, Associate Dean, Faculty of Economics and Social Sciences, Nottingham Trent University, England.

Fiona Williams Professor of Social Policy, Department of Sociology and Social Policy, University of Leeds, England.

Acknowledgements

The particular catalyst for this book was a twenty-four-hour seminar held at Keele University in May 1994 entitled 'Social Work in the New Age'. All the contributors to this book were participants. We would like to thank CCETSW for funding the seminar and the University of Keele for acting as hosts. It was a very rare experience indeed. The opportunity to think about and analyse in depth the nature and future(s) for social work is unusual. We would like to thank everyone involved, particularly Alex Scott and Jeff Hopkins whose suggestion it was in the first place and who kindly devised our Prologue. We would also like to thank Colin Smith for sorting out our various technologies and disks and Sue Hanson who helped bring it all together at the end.

Prologue

Once upon a time, on a grey, damp morning a poor tailor stood before the fitting mirror in his shop and looked at himself. He saw reflected in the mirror a weary and saddened man, whose pin-stripe trousers were shiny and whose patent leather shoes were dulled with wear. Sticking out of his waistcoat pocket was a pair of cutting scissors and draped around his neck was a tape measure. He sighed at the image in front of him. 'WHAT HAS BECOME OF ME?' he said to himself. 'What has happened to the life that once I led.' And he sobbed. Now it so happened that his words were carried up the chimney and out on to the street. There they fell into the path of a passing fairy who was moved to knock on his door and ask what was the matter. The tailor was not surprised at his visitor, for in truth nothing could have surprised him any more. He was a courteous man and invited the fairy into the kitchen at the back, where he sat her down and explained that it was such hard going being a tailor these days. She was a kindly fairy, but she knew little of the way things worked in the human world. When she asked him to explain about tailoring this is what he told her.

My job is to suit my customers. To help them look right in the eyes of others and to feel comfortable in themselves. The suits I provide are either tailored, which means I make them up from the cloth that I order specially, or they come ready made. Ready-made suits are cheaper. The tailored suits are usually of better quality and have a better fit. They are made up to the customer's instructions. But they come more expensive. The wider the range of material, the less the savings on the amount produced. And there are the extra costs for the time it takes me to make the material up and get the fitting right. Only a few customers can afford to have their suits made to measure in this way. The average customer buys the ready-made suit available from stock. I might have to make minor alterations so that it fits them a bit better. I sometimes make a small charge for this extra work.

The fairy, to whom all of this was a novelty, then asked where people who were not his customers got their suits from. The tailor, warming to her interest, explained that some of those people got their suits passed on from family or friends. Others went round to the charity shop; some out of necessity, others because they preferred the old-fashioned suits that no one made any more.

His problem, he explained, was that everyone now expected better quality. Even the people who come in to buy the ready made. This made all the suits more expensive. Not only because the material was more expensive in the first place, but all the quality checks that were made on it during the manufacturing process also had to be paid for. Nowadays he spent a lot of his time talking with customers, helping them understand why they couldn't get the suits they expected and then listening to their complaints.

The fairy asked if he couldn't just stretch the material to make it to go round. The tailor said that the material would then be strained and liable to tear, leaving big gaps in the suits. He would then spend all his time patching over the holes and this was not his trade. Anybody could get work as a patcher-over. They only needed to demonstrate that they could thread a needle competently. He was a tailor and he knew all about suits and how they were made; the history of fashion and how styles changed. He was able to help customers to make a considered choice when they were unsure or indecisive. He wanted people to value his suits and the service he provided. They would then come back to his shop and bring their friends.

The fairy was getting a bit bored by all this technical stuff for she did not really understand the niceties of tailoring. She never wore suits herself and thought that the affairs of human beings were not all that interesting. They seemed to take things so seriously. However, she was too polite to interrupt the tailor when he then went on to tell her about the impossible situation he found himself in.

Apparently, all sorts of people had been led to believe that they were now entitled to suits, and made-to-measure suits at that. The more people, the more the variety of shapes and sizes. This made it difficult to fit anybody up with the ready-wears. And the tailor could only afford the material for so many made to measure. He earned barely enough to live on, let alone put aside money to buy extra cloth. And if he sold all his suits straight away he would run out of stock very quickly. If customers then came into the shop and found it empty of suits they would be very annoyed, turn round and probably never come back again. So he always had to keep some suits back. He could show new customers the suits he had in and let them order from the stock and from pictures of other suits and promise to have their suit ready at some time in the future. People would then keep popping back in to see how their order was progressing. This gave the impression to passers-by that the shop was very busy. If he took a long time to write out the order, consulting all sorts of catalogues and ringing up suppliers, he could spin out the process even longer. But this, he said, wasn't tailoring, it was called shop management and although he had been told it was all very necessary, he didn't believe in it himself.

He then frowned, and said that his dear wife had suggested that he go back to the cloth manufacturers and tell them he wanted better material at cheaper prices, or he would not buy his cloth from them any more. This startled the fairy, for he was a gentle tailor and clearly not used to bullying other people. She was therefore reassured when he looked her straight in the eye and said, 'Or maybe I wish I could give up tailoring and try something different . . . like become a social worker.' And the fairy said to him, 'If you believe that, you really do believe in fairies', and granted his wish.

Chapter 1

Social theory, social change and social work

An introduction

Nigel Parton

Ever since the early 1970s social work in Britain has been highly contested and subject to a variety of public, political and professional debates and opprobrium often in the full glare of media attention (Franklin and Parton, 1991; Aldridge, 1994). However, recent years have witnessed new levels of uncertainty and change characterised by the 'destabilisation of an entire service system'. While this generates energy, excitement and new ideas, as Harding (1992) argues, it also generates high anxiety and stress for those involved, particularly if they have few opportunities to understand or influence it. 'The certainties of a professionally-driven, local authority-controlled service system no longer exist, and few people have a clear vision or experience of the potential alternatives' (Harding, 1992: 3).

At one level these uncertainties arise from the changes ushered in by the Children Act 1989, the National Health Services and Community Care Act 1990 and the Criminal Justice Act 1991, together with changes in the training of social workers, particularly the Diploma in Social Work (CCETSW, 1989). At another level, however, they reflect much wider and fundamental changes in the state, the economy and society more generally. What becomes evident is that the uncertainties which characterise contemporary social work can also be seen to characterise the nature and form of social transformations in Western societies more generally and which have been the focus of important debates in social theory.

The pace and intensity of change has been such that it has proved difficult to take stock of what is happening, what the implications might be and what futures might be opening up. It certainly seems that we are living through an important period of change in social work – in its priorities, organisation and day-to-day practices – and that its rationale and social locations are shifting in fundamental ways. Our central concern in this book is to analyse the changing nature of social work in the context of these wider social transformations and current debates in social theory. What can social work learn from these wider debates and how far can changes in contemporary social work be seen to exemplify particular instances of much wider transformations? However, the central question we are addressing, from our diverse perspectives, is how can we best understand and re-conceptualise contemporary social work and how can this then inform social work itself?

The other central theme running through the book is that conceptual and theoretical debate about social work and for social work has been severely lacking in recent years at a time when such debate is needed more than ever. The social-work academy has been marginalised. Yet, if social work is to think independently and reconstruct itself, academic debates, drawing on contemporary developments in social theory, are important. We should not be embarrassed by saying things that are troublesome and awkward and thereby open up the possibilities of seeing the world in different ways.

The purpose of this introductory chapter is threefold. It aims to provide a beginning framework for analysing the contemporary nature of social work and how this has changed over time. Second, it summarises some of the perspectives that have emerged in social theory in recent years for accounting for the nature of contemporary society and the key elements of social change. Reference will be made to perspectives associated with postmodernity, postmodernisation and post-Fordism. Finally, I will attempt to articulate, throughout the chapter, some of the key issues which social work is currently addressing and which figure centrally in the book.

THE CONTEMPORARY STATE OF SOCIAL WORK

The emergence of social work is associated with the transformations that took place from the mid-nineteenth century onwards around a series of anxieties about the family and the community more generally. Social work developed as a hybrid in the space, the 'social' (Donzelot, 1979), between the public and the private spheres and was produced by new relations between the law, administration, medicine, the school and the family. Social work was seen as a positive solution to a major problem posed for the liberal state;

namely, how can the state establish the health and development of family members who are weak and dependent, particularly children, while promoting the family as the 'natural' sphere for caring for those individuals and thus not intervening in all families (Hirst, 1981)? Social work developed at a midway point between individual initiative and the all-encompassing state, which would be in danger of taking responsibility for everyone's needs and hence undermining the responsibility and role of the family.

However, the space occupied by social work has always been complex as it is related to and, in part, dependent upon numerous other, more established discourses, particularly law, health/hygiene, psychiatry and education. As a consequence, defining the nature, boundaries and settings of social work, as distinct from other practices, has always been difficult. This difficulty may be one of social work's key defining and enduring characteristics (Stenson, 1993), for social work is in an essentially contested and ambiguous position. Most crucially, this ambiguity arises from its sphere of operation between civil society, with its allegiances to individuals and families, and the state in the guise of the court and its 'statutory' responsibilities. This ambiguity captures the central, but often submerged, nature of modern social work as it emerged from the late nineteenth century onwards. Social work occupied the space between the respectable and the dangerous classes, and between those with access to political and speaking rights and those who were excluded (Philp, 1979). Social work fulfils an essentially mediating role between those who are actually or potentially excluded and the mainstream of society.

As the twentieth century proceeded, the growth of modern social work was increasingly dependent upon its inter-relationships with the welfare state, which provided its primary rationale and legitimacy. As a result it mediated not only between the excluded and state agencies, but between other diverse state agencies and a wide range of private and voluntary philanthropic agencies and the diverse and overlapping discourses which informed and constituted them.

Thus the emergence and essential ambiguities of modern social work were closely related to the development of new forms of social regulation associated with the increased sophistication and complexity of modern society (Garland, 1985). These new forms of social regulation were characterised by notions of normalisation, discipline and surveillance (Foucault, 1977), and were originally associated with the development of the modern prison but were increasingly reflected in the school, the hospital, the family and the community. Modern systems of social regulation became blurred and wide-ranging (Cohen, 1985; A. Howe, 1994). The central focus of modern systems of regulation was the classification of the population based on the scientific claims of different experts in the 'psy' complex (Ingleby, 1985; Rose, 1985). Increasingly, modern societies regulated the population by sanctioning the knowledge claims and practices of the new human sciences – particularly medicine, psychiatry, psychology, criminology and social work.

The 'psy' complex refers to the network of ideas about the nature of human beings, their perfectibility, the reasons for their behaviour and the way they may be classified, selected and controlled. It aims to manage and improve individuals by the manipulation of their qualities and attributes and is dependent upon scientific knowledge and professional interventions and expertise. Human qualities are seen as measurable and calculable and thereby can be changed, improved and rehabilitated. The new human sciences had as their central aim the prediction of future behaviour.

The emergence of modern forms of social regulation was an integral element of the development of modernity. Modernity involved the recognition that human order is neither natural nor God-given (as in traditional or pre-modern society) but is essentially vulnerable and contingent. However, by the development and application of science it can be subject to human control. Contingency was discovered together with the recognition that things could be regular, repeatable and predictable and hence ordered. The vision of politicians joined with the practices of professionals and scientists to improve the world. The vision was of a hierarchical harmony reflected in the uncontested and incontestable pronouncements of reason. 'The modern, obsessively legislating, defining, structuring, segregating, classifying, recording and universalising state reflected the splendour of universal and absolute standards of truth' (Bauman, 1992: xiv).

Such assumptions were most evident in Britain, and elsewhere, with the establishment of the welfare state in the post-war period. The establishment of modern social work was a small, but significant, element of the 'welfarist' project as it developed in the twentieth century, and is most appropriately characterised as a 'bureau-profession' (Parry and Parry, 1979). The key innovations of 'welfarism' lay in the attempts to link the fiscal, calculative and bureaucratic capacities of the apparatus of the state to the government of social life (Rose and Miller, 1992). As a political rationality, 'welfarism' was structured by the wish to encourage national growth and well-being via the promotion of social responsibility and the mutuality of social risk and was premised on notions of social solidarity (Donzelot, 1988). 'Welfarism' rested on the twin pillars of Keynesianism and Beveridgianism.

A number of assumptions characterised 'welfarism'. The institutional framework of universal social services was seen as the best way of maximising welfare in modern society, and the nation state worked for the whole society and was the best way of progressing this. The social services were instituted for benevolent purposes, meeting social needs, compensating socially caused 'diswelfares' and promoting social justice. Their underlying functions were ameliorative, integrative and redistributive. Social progress would continue to be achieved through the agency of the state and professional intervention so that increased public expenditure, the cumulative extension of statutory welfare provision and the proliferation of government regulations backed by expert administration represented the main guarantors of equity, fairness and efficiency. Social scientific knowledge was given a pre-eminence in ordering the rationality of the emerging professions, which were seen as having a major contribution to developing individual and social welfare and thereby operationalising increasingly sophisticated mechanisms of social regulation.

Social work, in its modern emergence in the context of welfarism, was imbued with a considerable optimism, and it was believed that measured and significant improvements could be made in the lives of individuals and families by judicious professional interventions. The establishment of social service departments in the early 1970s reflected the belief of the Seebohm Report (1968) that social problems could be overcome via state intervention by professional experts with social-scientific knowledge and technical skills. It was imbued with a commitment to enhancing social citizenship through promoting greater equality and solidarity. Seebohm envisaged a progressive, universal service available to all and with wide community support. The notion of the generic professional social worker represented the hallmark and aspirations of the new service.

There seemed a consensus that social work was a positive development for all in the context of 'welfarism'. This consensus had a number of elements. It was assumed that the interests of the social worker, and hence the state, were similar to, if not the same as, the people they were trying to help. It was to be an essentially benign but paternalistic relationship. Interventions were not conceived as a potential source of antagonism between social workers and individuals and families. When an individual or a family required modification this would be through casework, help and advice, and if individuals did come into state care this was assumed to be in their – and the community's – interests. Interventions which had therapeutic intentions necessarily had therapeutic outcomes so that social work was allowed a large degree of independence and discretion to carry out its work. In the process, the essential ambiguities, tensions and uncertainties which lay at the core of its operations remained partially submerged.

The growth of social work and its claims to expertise during the twentieth century was characterised by its increasing allegiance to social casework. Not only did casework provide a systematic approach to practice, it also helped to unify internally an occupational group placed in a variety of locations and with diverse roles and responsibilities. Similarly, it provided an internally coherent knowledge base derived from psychodynamic theory and ego-psychology (Payne 1992; Pearson et al., 1988). While it would be incorrect to assume that casework dominated the thinking and practices of practitioners in a coherent and consistent manner, in Britain it provided a focus for professionalisation, and legitimated its location in the 'psy' complex more generally. Casework, however, provided a distinctive contribution in its claim to be concerned with the whole person and to provide particular personal skills in human relationships and an understanding of individuals and families. It provided a method for assessment and intervention and thereby appeared to legitimate social work and to overcome its essential ambiguities.

However, just at the point at which modern social work emerged in the early 1970s to play a significant part in the welfarist project, 'welfarism' itself was experiencing considerable strains and ultimately crises. A combination of slow economic growth, increases in inflation and a growth in social disorder and indiscipline undermined the central economic and social pillars of welfarism and the political consensus which supported it. In the process, the various human sciences and the bureau-professionals who operated and applied them were seen to be found inadequate for the problems that were presented. At one level the criticisms levelled at social work from the mid-1970s can be understood as a specific case of the neo-liberal approach which has dominated government in recent years, in terms of an antagonism towards public expenditure on state welfare; an increasing emphasis on self-help and family support; the centrality of individual responsibility, choice and freedom; and an extension of the commodification of social relations. However, this would be simplistic. Social work has failed to meet the aspirations expected of it and vocal criticism has come from a variety of quarters, including the left, feminists and anti-racists, from a variety of user groups, other professional and community interests, as well as the anti-welfarist right (Clarke, 1993). Increasingly, social work and, in particular, social service departments were seen as costly, ineffective, distant and oppressive, leaving the user powerless and without a voice.

What has emerged is a reconstruction of social work and the agencies in which it operates which is very consistent with the central themes characterising the reconstruction of welfare more generally. First, there is a particular emphasis on market principles primarily through the 'quasi-market' (Le Grand, 1990; Le Grand and Bartlett, 1993), which has a number of features: a split between purchasing and providing responsibilities; a concern for services to be based upon need and the assessment of risk rather than historic demand and service levels; the delegation of authority for budgetary control; and the pursuit of choice through provider competition.

Second, there is the emergence of 'government by contract' (Stewart, 1993b): the introduction of contractual rather than hierarchical accountability whereby relationships within and between welfare organisations should be specific and formally spelt out and costed. Similarly, at the consumer/professional interface the nature of the relationships and the focus of work should be formally spelt out in a contract.

Third, there is the development of more responsive and often flatter organisations where responsibilities and decisions are devolved down and where the user/consumer is more directly involved. Notions of enabling, decentralisation and empowerment are seen as of significance and the nature of professionalism shifts. Various performance indicators, outcome measures and business plans are introduced.

Such developments cannot be reduced to the impact of market-orientated approaches alone. 'Welfare pluralism' and 'mixed-economies of welfare' are summary terms often used to indicate more fluid and fragmented arrangements whereby social work, now often called 'social care', is provided by voluntary agencies, private organisations and community initiatives, and where other non-professional staff are seen as more appropriate particularly in the provision of practical services.

In the process, the role and practices of managers become crucial. It is managers, as opposed to professionals, who are seen as the key brokers in the new network (Clarke *et al.*, 1994; Cutler and Waine, 1994), and notions of management frame and supplant the central activities of the professionals themselves and the forms of knowledge they draw upon. There is a clear move away from approaches to social work which are based on therapeutic models and which stress the significance of casework. Social workers, reconstituted as care managers, are required to act as coordinators of care packages for individuals on the basis of an assessment of need or risk. A distinction is made between the purchaser and the provider which effectively splits the traditional social-work role. Care managers crucially require skills in: the assessment of need and risk; co-ordinating packages of care; costing and managing of the budgets for services; and monitoring and evaluation of progress and outcome. There is a renewed emphasis on inter-agency coordination and multi-disciplinary joint working which has to recognise the increasingly fragmented nature of services and expertise.

The emergence of child protection as a central activity for social workers underlines the centrality of social workers in providing social assessments of 'risk' and 'dangerousness' (Parton, 1991), but which recognises there are various interests and rights at stake – particularly those of the child and parent(s). Decisions in child care are now carried out in a more legalised context where the need for forensic evidence is prioritised. The assessment and management of risk and separation of the high risk from the rest become crucial, so that both harm to children and unwarrantable interventions in the family can be avoided. Similarly, in recognising that different people have diverse interests and that situations and risks may be judged differently in different circumstances and according to different criteria – for example, arising from different gender or ethnic backgrounds – the monolithic notions of knowledge and power are opened up. It is recognised that cultural relativities are important and that professionals may not always know best.

It is possible, therefore, to identify a complex reconstitution of generic social work and the unified model of the personal social services. A number of elements are evident. First, increased specialisation around client groups and the separation of assessment and care management from the work of direct service provision. Second, the concentration of professionally qualified staff in certain roles and responsibilities – again around assessment and care management – while an increasing number of services are provided by fewer and unqualified staff. Third, the changes attempt to shift the power relationship between the client – now consumer or service user – and the professional. While the main vehicle for this in the community care sphere is primarily by marketisation and commodification, in the child-care field it is via increased legalism and accountability to the court (Langan, 1993b). Notions of management become central.

No longer are social workers constituted as caseworkers drawing on their therapeutic skills in human relationships, but as care managers assessing need and risk and operationalising packages of care where notions of monitoring and review are central. In effect, casework has been reconstituted as counselling and a new, diverse and fast-growing occupation has developed. While some may be full-time and have a background in social work, this is not necessarily so, and many counsellors work on a part-time, independent or fee-only basis. The net result is that activities and skills previously seen as key to social work are now more likely to be included in a package as and when required and provided by specialist counsellors in various guises.

TOWARDS THE (POST)MODERN?

Thus it seems that social work is experienced as being subject to increasing diversity, uncertainty, fragmentation, ambiguity and change – themes which have been the focus of attention in social theory and which have been seen as pointing to the possible emergence of the postmodern. Recent years have witnessed an increasing interest in understanding changes in welfare in terms of postmodernity (see Williams, 1992; Burrows and Loader, 1994; Taylor-Gooby, 1994) and some writers have applied such approaches to social work in particular (see Rojek et al., 1988; McBeath and Webb, 1991; Sands and Nuccio, 1992; Pardeck et al., 1994; Parton, 1994a; Parton, 1994b; Pozatek, 1994; Howe, 1994).

Notions of postmodernity have essentially developed from immanent critiques of modernity. 'Modernity', as a summary term, refers to the cluster of social, economic and political systems which emerged in the West with the Enlightenment. Unlike the pre-modern era, modernity recognised that human order is neither natural nor God-given but is vulnerable and contingent. However, by the development and application of science, nature could be subject to human control.

The distinguishing features of modernity are: the understanding of history as having a definite and progressive direction; the attempt to develop universal categories of experience, representation and explanation; the idea that reason can provide a basis for all activities; and that the nation state could coordinate and advance such developments for the whole society. The guiding principle of modernity was the search to establish reliable foundations for generalisable knowledge, policy and practice. Modernity may be defined in terms of the aspiration to reveal the central truth(s) about the world but recognises that truth does not reside on the surface of things but is hidden by appearances. 'Defining modernity in the terms of uncovering, of ripping away the layers of disguise, of disclosing and realising the premise or threat of the future by moving on and through where we are now, enables us to reconcile the various sides of modernity' (Boyne and Rattansi, 1990: 8). The two key elements of modernity were the progressive fusion of scientific objectivity and politico-economic rationality.

Increasingly it is being suggested that we are now living through a period of such fundamental and complex transformations in the social, economic, cultural and technological spheres that we are witnessing something quite different – the emergence of the postmodern. At the same time there is considerable debate about the significance of the developments and whether they form a distinct break with the past. Some have argued that the changes have been overstated or oversignified (Clarke, 1991); others, that the changes, at the economic and political level, merely represent new forms of class relations in the pursuit of profit and exploitation (Callinicos, 1989; Jameson, 1991); and others that what we are experiencing is not a distinct break with the past but a period of 'late' or 'high' modernity (Giddens, 1990, 1991). Contributors to this book vary in their respective positions on these debates and how significant they see them for both explaining the nature of contemporary change and their significance for social work. What we agree on is that they capture the sense of current pace and change; draw attention to the importance of difference and diversity; underline the significance of a variety of new political strategies and social movements; and take seriously the level of critique and destabilisation directed at a whole range of previous assumptions, received wisdoms and practices.

Notions of postmodernity, postmodernisation and post-Fordism serve to describe the central features and processes of the various global transformations taking place since the early 1960s. For while production was the key determining influence of modern society – the way it is organised for production considerably influences the political, cultural and social spheres – this is no longer necessarily the case. Postmodernisation involves a reversal of determinacy so that the fragments of a hyperdifferentiating culture disrupt and deconstruct areas of social structure which were previously seen as central and immovable – particularly social class. Processes of consumption and changes in culture increasingly impact upon the market and hence production. There is a massive compression of time and space, particularly via the pervasive impact of information technology and the growth of media (Harvey, 1989). Markets become saturated and consumers begin to exercise choice, while production systems are forced into structural changes that allow flexible responses to new and different consumer demands (Crook *et al.*, 1992).

The growth of new technology allows for a number of changes in the organisation of work in contemporary society: the expansion of the service sector by the reduction of labour required for production; the reduction of capital costs of production increases the possibilities for self-employment; and new opportunities are opened up for alternative forms of organisation which do not rely on hierarchy, the bureaucracy and the traditional professional and occupational divides. Notions of flexibility and fragmentation in both production and organisation are increasingly evident – what are referred to as flexible accumulation or post-Fordism.

It is suggested that if Fordism was represented by notions of mass production, mass consumption, modernist cultural forms and the mass public provision of welfare, then post-Fordism is characterised by an emerging coalition between flexible production, differentiated and segmented consumption patterns, postmodern cultural forms and a restructured welfare state (Loader and Burrows, 1994). As Fiona Williams has suggested previously:

At a simple level the application of the post-Fordist analysis to welfare suggests that changes in the organisation of both production and consumption in the wider economy have influenced and even been reproduced within the provision of welfare: mass production to flexible production; mass consumption to diverse patterns of consumption; production-led to consumer-led; from mass, universal needs met by monolithic, bureaucratic/ professional-led provision to the diversity of individual needs met by welfare pluralism, quasi-markets, reorganised welfare work and consumer sovereignty.

(Williams, 1994: 49)

Central to the changes are moves to create the flexible organisation of different work patterns, lines of accountability and forms of decision-making. The emphasis is upon strategic management, quality control processes, responsiveness, creativity, teamwork, managerial decentralisation, flexibility of labour and numerical flexibility. It is argued that a key element in the complex and diverse re-conceptualisation and restructuring of state welfare is a new role for management. The growth of managerialism in recent years is seen as the connecting thread linking markets, partnerships, an emphasis on customers and the recomposition of the labour force (Taylor-Gooby and Lawson, 1993). It is transforming the relationships of power, culture, control and accountability (Clarke *et al.*, 1994). The new manager is key to operationalising the increasingly complex and fragmented organisational grids.

The development of flexible organisations and new technology allows for the transfer of productive capacity, or service provision, out of the core organisations. A variety of consequences follow. Permanent full-time workers in the core organisation need new training as their personal skills and abilities assume increasing importance; middle management is released and specialised services contracted out on a need basis; labour-intensive production (or service provision) requiring high levels of supervision is external-ised; and in many instances the process of decentralisation goes as far as destructuring the core organisation itself into a looser arrange-ment. Around core organisations are emerging networks of smaller-scale units with a variety of contractual arrangements with other organisations and with their own employees. These include small professional and technical organisations operating on a fee-for or consultancy service with a pronounced petty-entrepreneurial char-acter; specialist craftwork shops producing niche-market products or complex services supplied to core organisations on a contractual basis; labour-intensive 'sweat-shops' employing in the secondary labour market on a relatively insecure basis; entrepreneurial contract suppliers of various manual services such as cleansing and catering and who also tend to employ in the secondary labour market; and beyond these manual homeworkers who are invariably subject to the greatest insecurity and lowest material reward.

While these changes in the social, economic, cultural and technological spheres are of considerable importance and have clearly had an impact on the organisation and nature of contemporary social work, it is important that we do not restrict our analysis to these areas alone. For in many respects it is developments in the aesthetic, intellectual and epistemological which capture the crucial elements of the postmodern condition.

The notion of postmodernity recognises that we now inhabit a world which has become disorientated, disturbed and subject to doubt. The pursuit of order and control, the promotion of calculability, the belief in progress, science and rationality and other features intrinsic to modernity are increasingly being undermined by a simultaneous range of negative conditions and experiences and the persistence of chance and the threat of indeterminacy. Postmodernity is characterised by the fragmentation of modernity into forms of institutional pluralism, marked by variety, difference, contingency, relativism and ambivalence – all of which modernity sought to overcome. It is this constant and growing questioning of modern resolutions that has been diagnosed as symptomatic of the existence of the postmodern condition. Modernity becomes visible only from the moment that it distances itself from us and thereby becomes socially and ontologically unsettling.

It is suggested that the crucial elements for capturing the nature of postmodernity is as a form of historical consciousness which has developed in response to the problems with modernity (Bauman, 1991, 1992; Heller and Feher, 1988; Smart, 1993). It is presented as a way of relating to the consequences of modernity – the unfulfilled promises, the thwarted aspirations and the inherent dilemmas which now have to be addressed without the belief in rational resolutions. Problems cannot be overcome by quick technical fixes and there are no final resolutions to the dilemmas and difficulties encountered in social life.

Even those who are highly critical of analyses that argue we are moving towards the postmodern recognise the claim that we have experienced a considerable loss of confidence in science and experts as offering the routes to solving economic, social and human problems (Taylor-Gooby, 1994). Increasingly, notions of ambi-valence, contingency, risk and reflexivity are seen as characteristic of our contemporary condition.

Postmodern perspectives put particular emphasis on the con-temporary significance of fragmentation, difference, relativity and plurality, and the liberation of diverse identities. There are important points of connection amongst postmodern theorists in their discus-sions of the decentring of the subject, the rejection of grand narratives, the espousal of the local and the centrality of language not simply in representing reality but in constituting it.

Thus a central postmodern tenet is the refusal to prescribe some discourses as essentially true, and to proscribe others as irredeem-ably false. For a key postmodern operation is that of deconstruction whereby phenomena are continually interrogated, evaluated, dis-rupted and overturned. Nothing is taken for granted and phenomena are always likely to be subject to critique and changed. It pluralises and politicises the processes of reaching a verdict in areas which were previously taken for granted and closed off and has the effect of politicising all areas of personal and social life. The operation of deconstruction is evident both in a number of chapters in this book and also in terms of day-to-day practice in the ways I have suggested earlier. However, the processes of deconstruction imply that social work itself, certainly in ways we have previously come to understand and experience it, disappears or, at least, is reconstructed in quite new ways. Thus, while potentially quite liberating, postmodern perspectives are also potentially disabling and nihilistic. However, they do seem to speak in part to the current state of social work.

If social work is being deconstructed and reconstructed in terms of care management, counselling, social care and child protection, for example, how far can we be said to be still talking about social work? Where postmodern perspectives can be seen to be particularly unhelpful is in their reluctance to articulate the criteria for judging improvement and coming close to saying 'anything goes'. This is not a defensible position and not one taken up in this book.

What we do argue, and numerous examples are offered, is that perhaps we have a wider scope for creativity and self-determination than we often assume and that things can be changed. Inevitably, however, we have to assume responsibility with others for shaping and reconstructing our futures. The 'vertigo of relativity' is the corollary of increasing choice and questioning.

What the earlier part of this chapter attempted to demonstrate was that, ever since the moment of its modern emergence in the nineteenth century, social work has always been an ambiguous activity, characterised, in part, by a tension between the forces of fragmentation and diversity and attempts to pursue occupational coherence and professional legitimacy (Clarke, 1993). Through much of our recent history these tensions and ambiguities have been masked and hidden but have now come to characterise social work in a period of rapid change.

We cannot assume, however, that the nature of our current experiences is simply our old ambiguities, tensions and contradictions come back to haunt us. This is unlikely to be the case. For while ambiguity may constitute the essential nature of contemporary social work, it is more important than ever that we honestly and coherently articulate the various elements and developments that make this up. This is the central agenda which each contributor, with their particular perspectives and area of substantive concern, attempts to address in this book. We may then be in a better position to influence and (re)fashion our futures. It is open to question, however, whether this is most appropriately conceptualised in terms of social work and, if it is, how this relates to what went before.

While the focus is primarily social-work policy and practice, all of the chapters, some explicitly, raise issues in relation to the nature and implications for social-work education and more particularly the role of theory and the academy in the social-work enterprise and vision(s) for the future. The book brings together a range of academics involved in various aspects of research and teaching in relation to social work. All are committed to developing critical analyses and perspectives in different areas of the social sciences, for the purpose of understanding social work and making a positive contribution to policy, practice and education. The book is organised in a way which initially addresses themes and questions of wide concern to social work and then analyses certain substantive areas in more detail.

Chapter 2

Social work through the looking glass

Jeff Hopkins

The modernist approach to social welfare is underpinned by a belief in the worth and possibility of material progress through the application of scientific method to economic and social affairs. This view was promoted by the professional intellectual classes who first achieved status in the nineteenth century and whose relative decline in influence during recent years has led to speculation about the end of modernism. Their demise is associated with a more general loss of faith in finding rational solutions to the problems presently confronting society.

The history of social work is afforded little more than a footnote in the development of the professions. However, it is the thesis of this chapter that the development of social work has been closely bound to the fate of those liberal members of the professional classes who took a benign view towards those less fortunate than themselves and served as the mentors of social work. The development of professional social work in the United Kingdom has been closely tied to the fate of those mentors within government and the civil service.

This chapter opens with a review of the beginnings of modernism as recounted through the emergence of a particular class; it then illustrates how the fortune of that class was mirrored by developments in social work, drawing on examples from the past. The chapter concludes with an analysis of present events and speculation as to future developments.

THE EMERGENCE OF THE PROFESSIONAL INTELLECTUAL CLASSES

Perkin (1969) provides a useful account of the origins of modernism in the nineteenth century when he describes the emergence of a new class with a source of income that freed them from patronage and financial obligation. Using the definition of class as determined principally by source of income, he argues that

> Doctors and officials receive incomes which differ less from each other than they do from rent, capital or wages. The first profession was that of the clergy, whose income, significantly, was called a 'living'; an income set aside by the laity, not as a reward for their service – which, once incumbent in their living, they were free except in conscience to supply or omit – but a guaranteed income to enable them to perform their office. The second and third were those of law and medicine, in which fees might first seem to bear some relation in detail to piece rates and aggregate in profits. Yet fees too were not (in theory) fixed by competition, but by the value set by the profession, and accepted by society, on services which the client could not judge and had therefore to take on trust. All true professions are characterised by expert, esoteric service demanding integrity in the purveyor and trust in the client and the community, and by non-competitive reward in the form of a fixed salary or standard and unquestioned fee.
>
> (Perkin, 1969: 253–4)

It was their freedom from the struggle for income that emancipated professionals as a class from the control of the laity.

With little or no pecuniary interest in the outcome of their work, the professional men, and later in the twentieth century professional women, were free to make informed and objective judgement based on expertise rather than personal advantage. Their success was measured by their influence in assisting others in the resolution of the problems and dilemmas confronting them.

> Doctors, lawyers, civil servants, engineers, scientists, social workers, teachers and professional thinkers brought their disinterested intelligence to bear upon the problems of the nineteenth century. They were not necessarily superior, morally or intellectually, to their fellows in other classes, but they had a professional interest in disinterestedness and intelligence. It was their interest to 'deliver the goods' which they purveyed; expert service and the objective solution of society's problems, whether disease, legislation, administration, material construction, the nature of matter, social misery, education, or social, economic and political theory.
>
> (Perkin, 1969: 260)

It was through their trained expertise, confirmed by qualification, that professionals justified their new-found status and power. Recruitment into the professions was based on the examination of the candidates' understanding of the knowledge base. This could only be judged by other professionals in the chosen field. Access to membership was through a self-regulating process. The new professional institutes that sprang up were preoccupied with professional examinations.

Peer-judged entry was subsequently absorbed by the state itself through reforms in entry to the civil service. These in turn led to the modernisation of government through the process of inquiry, report, legislation, administration and inspection. It was the professional intellectuals who developed statistical records as the language of industrialisation, were members of the flourishing statistical societies and provided these with access to government returns and information. Their political masters came to depend on them for information and look to them for 'objective' recommendations based on the evidence submitted. Perkin argues that the demand for expert solutions to the emerging social problems was met and manipulated by the professional intellectuals. Whilst the 'entrepreneurial ideal' was satisfied by minimalist regulations, the new class pressed on with the expanding bureaucratic, centralised, interventionist state of Victorian practice.

Although a more recent offspring, social work until recently shared many of the characteristics of its class parentage. Social workers remained free from any pecuniary interest in the outcome of their work, their activity was underpinned by a knowledge base in the social sciences, their expertise in assisting others to resolve their social problems and dilemmas was recognised as of value to society, and qualification was based on peer judgement of the candidates' ability, diligence and expertise in their chosen field. They also had faith that they were working in some modest, but immediate, way towards the general improvement of society.

The inter-relationship between social workers and their professional intellectual mentors is explored below. The illustrations are followed by a discussion of future developments. This draws on an account of the parallel struggle of professionals in the Health Service to resist attempts to subjugate their status and authority.

The Charity Organisation Society

Although established in 1869, the Society for Organising Charitable Relief and Repressing Mendicity held its first meeting in March 1870.

The movement that gave form to the Charity Organisation Society (COS) in the late nineteenth century was a reactionary movement to secure the betterment of the poor through social advancement. It attributed the failure of the market economy to deliver the expected harmonious and balanced society to the immorality and lack of self-discipline of the impoverished classes. They were held to be responsible for their situation. The principle of the movement was personal effort – voluntary effort on the part of the charitable, to encourage the voluntary effort of the poor (through the offices of organised charity run by the voluntary committee and volunteers). The movement derived its vigour from the affirmation of its commitment to the 'scientific approach'.

The mentors of the COS were those members of the emerging professional intellectual class who took a liberal attitude towards the plight of the poor. They promoted the claims of scientific thinking, and believed that the application of the 'disinterested intelligence' approach towards the administration of charitable relief would resolve the problem of poverty and relieve the human misery associated with it. It was they who discovered the facts about social conditions, were disturbed by them, theorised and formulated plans to remedy them and who, within a civil service based on expertise and selection by merit, eventually implemented the machinery of reform.

The faith in modernism extended to the ranks of local middle-class men of standing in business and the professions, who had assumed the role of the 'urban squire', and with it a paternal responsibility for the welfare and discipline of the working-class poor. The nature of the social movement defined by Seed (1973) is complex. It was at once an emotive reaction against declining values and a faith in scientific reasoning. It was pursued with moral vigour and the absolute conviction that its members knew what was in the best interests of the poor themselves and of society. 'Its members made no prior assumption about those who applied for charity. They investigated every case systematically and distinguished between the helpable and those who were not' (Seed, 1973: 40).

'The first publications of the COS in 1870 were on the organization of district charities, house to house visiting, and included six District Committee papers containing bye-laws, forms and statements of principles' (Woodroofe, 1966: 42). Woodroofe describes the forms and report books issued in which uniform and confidential records of each case were written. There was also a file of press reports on noted cases of imposters and others. A spate of occasional papers was also unleashed which covered, amongst other things, instruction in the arts of district visiting and casework. The focus on administration is confirmed by Gilbert (1966):

> The COS was not a relief society in the ordinary sense of the word, 'but an organising society desirous of promoting the most effectual assistance for those in distress, and of creating at the same time a great co-operative association of charities'.
>
> (1966: 52)

Techniques were codified around the application, the interview, the investigation and the case committee, all monitored through the maintenance of written reports and records. In this way each case could be known and studied individually yet disposed of in the light of common principles.

Within the differentiated tasks set out in the COS it is possible to identify the emergence of roles that would become familiar features of social work. The casework assessment method involved the completion of administrative enquiries, the preparation of proposals based on the evidence of 'witnesses interviewed' and the submission of the proposals to the committee for the deployment of charitable funds.

Caseworkers also acted as brokers. They were expected to have a knowledge of local charitable sources and their boundaries of eligibility, together with policies and practices of local employers and the guardians. Much attention was addressed to the cooperation between these agencies.

'Moral' support was provided to the recipient of charity through the development of a *beneficent relationship*. A volunteer of standing and character was assigned to the case and their personal interest was expected to be an encouragement to the applicant. Amongst the volunteers, who visited the beneficiaries in their homes, were to be found the wives and daughters of members of the committee. Smith comments that activist volunteers were advised to become guardians or county councillors or promote the election of desirable candidates.

From its inception the COS committees had *paid employees*,

usually respectable men from the lower middle classes, to check out the applicants and collect loans. They were variously identified as collectors, enquirers or enquiry agents. However, in 1883 the COS accepted the principle of employed secretaries, in spite of reservations that they would supersede or lessen the need for the volunteers.

The distinction between education and training became blurred. By the end of the century training volunteers had become an important part of the work of the Secretary and the Districts Committee. Studies addressed the understanding and removal of poverty by raising the people to independence. It was assumed that technical methods had neither academic respectability nor a teachable content. Eventually the shortage of funds led to the transfer of training into the new Department of Social Science and Administration at the London School of Economics.

> With the transfer of what had begun as a professional education plan for social workers, to an academic institution without a clear understanding of the differences involved, only one result could obtain; the professional aspects would become less important and the theoretical more important.
>
> (Smith, 1965: 59)

Thus the modernisation of social welfare provision began with a preoccupation with efficient administration. This reflected the interest of the original mentors. Social-work method was an incidental part of the administrative process.

The Curtis Report (1946)

By the mid-1930s a consensus had been achieved in the centre of British politics in favour of a mixed economy. The Depression of the 1930s had led to the clamour of businessmen for protection from the rigours of the free market. Keynesian economics offered the opportunity for state intervention to stabilise the vagaries of the market economy.

Whatever their politics, the younger generation of graduates took the possibility of social planning seriously. Titmuss (1954) describes how the status of the political and social scientists rose during the war that followed. The management of the nation at war was accepted as an overriding necessity. The extension of the powers of the state, emerging piecemeal through the 1930s, was reinforced by this wartime activity. He argues that the tendency for administrative considerations to overrule other considerations continued after the Second World War, as social and economic policy became a matter for intelligent participation and conscious direction.

In March 1945 the Curtis Committee was set up to consider the evidence regarding, and make recommendations for, those children who were overlooked in the general preoccupation with plans for post-war reconstruction. The Report of the Care of Children Committee was published in 1946. The main theme of the Report was 'the shocking ignorance about the young among the majority of adults in charge of these children. Worst off of all are the children in the workhouse' (Curtis Committee, 1946: 119).

The committee found that one of the great difficulties in the way of coordination was a traditional inter-departmental antagonism which was sometimes thinly veiled by changes in organisation. It was also felt that administration had become too remote and that it was imperative that the personal element be introduced in the ambit of the local authority. The Report proposed the establishment of an *ad hoc* committee within the local authority which would co-opt experts and protect the interests of the deprived child. The Home Office was to provide an Inspectorate to monitor the activities of the Children's Department from central government. The personal nature of the service was emphasised. 'No office staff dealing with them can do what we want done' (Curtis Committee, 1946: 441).

The committee envisaged that a Children's Officer, probably female, would be appointed as Executive Officer and that she would maintain personal contact with each child. The committee stressed that the interests of the deprived child should come second to none. The way for the new department to achieve authority and status within the affairs of the local authority lay in the personal qualities and qualifications of those appointed Children's Officers. It was the view of the committee that the Children's Officer should be highly qualified academically, if possible a graduate who also had a social science diploma.

A clerk was to be appointed and charged with administering the arrangements established by the Children's Officer and ensuring that administrative procedures were in line with those required by local government. The immediate priority was the boarding out in foster homes of children in institutional care.

The government was surprised by the post-war demand for places on social-work courses. The Education Act 1944 had made it possible to undertake training with state support in the form of a student grant. This opened the doors to men and women alike, with the result that a flood of older men and women went straight from the armed services into the universities and on to the social science courses.

A review of social work at the beginning of 1946 conducted by Younghusband (1947) claimed that social workers remained concerned with economic need, although decreasingly so. Social science courses still offered the liberal view of 'man' in society, including a study of ethics, local and central government and social economics. Where psychology was offered it was academic and concerned with the abnormal, with little focus on normal growth and behaviour. For the bulk of their lectures social science students 'sat in' on courses for other degree students. Only five out of eighteen social science departments attempted to teach the theory and practice of social work.

The Curtis Report sharpened the focus of social-work training. A group of Training Inspectors were charged with developing the courses for Boarding Out Officers. These courses were postgraduate, and students were expected to have a social science qualification. The tutors appointed initially were all psychiatric social workers and the psychoanalytic ethos pervaded throughout training both on the courses and within the Inspectorate.

Thus a new profession of child care emerged at the behest of the Curtis Committee. Their Report marks a significant rise in the influence of the 'hands-on' practitioner within the framework of a statutory service.

The Seebohm Report (1968)

The Report of the Committee on Local Authority and Allied Personal Social Services in 1968 provides evidence of the increasing influence of the social-work professions on the shaping of social welfare provision.

The Report was, itself, the product of a long and close association between the social workers and their mentors within government, the civil service and the universities. The relationship was mutually productive in that it advanced the intellectual and professional base of social work and ensured that developments were informed by a high level of expertise.

The post-war period had been one in which change was essentially incremental and derived primarily from developments in practice.

Developments in social work were seen as part of the general progress of welfare provision. The service had become 'profession-led', with qualified social workers claiming to be managed by their 'own people', if managed at all. Administrators were seen as reactive to developments rather than instrumental in bringing about positive change.

The rapid expansion of social work in local government during the 1960s led to the movement of qualified social workers into the organisational hierarchy as team leaders, thereby permeating professional influence throughout the organisational structure, particularly in the area of child care. The Home Office initiated a programme of short management courses for child care team leaders. These programmes were devised by Home Office Inspectors, Children's Officers and child care tutors, and seen as a helpful contribution to professional development.

The professional associations within social work now came together within the Standing Conference of Social Workers to advocate a broad-based family service. The work was undertaken by a small group, mostly associated with the National Institute of Social Work. They advocated an enquiry to cover all the social-work services within local authorities and, by the use of memoranda and personal contacts with ministers, they succeeded in achieving a small independent Committee of Enquiry under the Chairman of the National Institute of Social Work, Frederick Seebohm.

The findings were very much a promulgation of the view that the common elements of social work in the different settings were more important than the elements that distinguished them. It was argued that it was in the interests of social workers themselves to have a wider range of cases offering a variety of interests and the opportunity for wider professional development.

The family service advocated in the Seebohm Report was to be based in area offices with the intention to forge the identity with local communities and to encourage mutual aid, especially in the inner city areas. The committee called for the maximum participation of clients, individuals and groups in planning, organisation and provision of social services. The proposed arrangement brought together the social-work services of the local authority Children's, Welfare and Health Departments.

Hall (1976) points out that the evidence on specialisation presented to the committee was, on balance, in favour of continued specialisation on existing or new lines. The decision to recommend a reduction in specialisation, against the weight of the views presented, was particularly contentious. Perhaps more than any other recommendation it armed critics with 'evidence' that the primary aim of the enquiry was to develop a united social-work profession. The Report advocated a professional leadership of the new Social Services Department,

> No single profession in Local Government at present combines the ideal range of skills which will be required of the Head of Department . . . most Directors of Social Service Departments were expected to be qualified in social work, who have received training in management and administration at appropriate points in their careers, or administrators with qualifications in Social Work.
>
> (Seebohm Committee, 1968: para 620)

In the successful political lobbying that followed the publication of the Report the Association of Child Care Officers and the Association of Children's Officers were particularly influential (Hopkins, 1969). However, the legislation was delayed.

Richard Crossman (1977), the Minister at the Department of Health and Social Security, describes the reluctance of the Home Secretary to surrender the Children's Services, and the personal agreement he reached that the move would not take place until the Home Secretary moved out of that office. The National Health Service Green Paper, the Proposals for Local Government Reorganisation and the Local Authorities Social Services Bill were all published within a fortnight towards the end of the life of the Labour government. No financial implications were implied, as this would delay the procedure.

The close relationship between their mentors and those employed in social work during the post-war period served the advancement of professional interests within government and the administration of social welfare. It also secured the advancement of the professionals themselves. This was not to last.

THE CHALLENGE TO MODERNISM AND SOCIAL WORK

The lack of 'progress' in the redistribution of power in society was exposed during the period of social protest that marked the late 1960s and early 1970s. The disillusion brought to an end the optimism of the post-war years. The counter-culture of intellectual libertarianism within the universities merged with radical sociology to show how existing political and social institutions were being used to label and package the poor and disarm them from demanding their rights. It was seen as deliberate challenge by the New Left to those who sought to mitigate the personal disadvantages inherent in institutional structures without challenging the basis of the authority that sustained them. The professions were seen as no more than servants of the establishment. Social workers supported individuals who were trapped in poverty, ill health or crime by the political, social and economic structures and by doing so provided only expedient palliatives. Social work with individuals was itself an obstacle to change.

It was expected by the radical academics that the new generation of social workers would, in turn, radicalise the social-work agencies and the structures in which they operated. Social-work training courses were themselves part of the movement sweeping through universities. Student social workers demanded participation in course planning and the management of courses. The new level of consciousness of the political context of social work led to a change in direction within social-work training. Community action was restored to the programmes and psychoanalytic-based casework no longer commanded respect and was marginalised. Theoretical models were introduced which reframed the personal problems experienced by clients as a response to their present rather than past circumstances. As a result, social work surrendered all professional claim to a clinical expertise.

When the colleges did push their way directly into the agencies, however, it was primarily to expand the number of student placements and to provide brief training for placement supervisors. This in turn led to the appointment of training officers to manage placement provision and the secondment arrangements for their own staff as well as to develop in-service training. The machinery was in place to expand employment-based, non-qualifying training.

THE DEMISE OF MODERNISM AND SOCIAL WORK

Faced with both a stagnant economy and rising inflation, the Tory government of 1979 attempted its own radical solutions to the problems facing it. Economic priority was switched from the pursuit of full employment to the control of inflation. Curtailing public expenditure was seen as necessary to control inflation. The welfare state had become the most rapidly growing sector of public spending in the 1970s and was therefore the prime target.

The critical attention paid to institutions of the welfare state reflected the view that public services were inefficient; that large-scale bureaucracies inevitably led to empire-building among the bureaucrats; and that they had become run for the benefit of staff rather than citizens or taxpayers. These views were reinforced by constant media attention on the casualties of 'blundering', and the image projected of social work was of a service dogged by controversy.

The desire to dismantle the provisions of the welfare state led to an attack on those who sustained them, this time from the New Right. Within the Cabinet itself liberal colleagues were dismissed as 'wets'. Particular invective was reserved for those associated with the socialist 'enemy' within the state, including the 'radical sociologists' who had sparked the call for structural change in the early 1970s. The attack was broadened out to a challenge to the concept of society itself, and social scientists were branded as political agitators.

No longer impressed by the quality of dispassionate intelligence, the conviction politicians pursued their own radical agendas. In these circumstances representations by liberal professional intellectuals were more likely to be counter-productive than helpful. Representations by social workers on behalf of client groups were dismissed as whinging.

The participation politics of the early 1970s was replaced by dynamic management in the 1980s. The entrepreneur was introduced into the public services, charged with dealing with the 'feather-bedding' of the unions and the professionals, and was to make the services 'lean and mean'. The underlying drive of the government was to bring order to the confusion of social and economic change through the re-assertion of discipline. A new wave of 'dynamic' managers rolled through the public services whose task was to contain budgets and to ensure that staff fell into line.

Consumer choice replaced equity as the tenet by which service was judged. Clients became customers, and the relationship between service provider and service user became a contractual one. More weight was given to the roles of assessor and broker than that of providing 'support'. The nature of the relationship between worker and client, on which the development of the professional identity was constructed, became an incidental part of the business between them.

The present restraints on public expenditure and changes in

employment practices threaten the continued employment of permanent salaried staff. Internal markets are being created within the agencies and different sections of the organisation are identified as cost centres. The culture of service agreements extends the control of service users over the arrangements provided to meet their needs. The present intention is that departments become purchasers of services from independent suppliers with only a rump of statutory services provided directly by the departments themselves. The discipline of the market, the contract culture and, latterly, the introduction of performance-related pay, increased the level of accountability to the 'laity'. The security and level of income are increasingly determined by criteria that have little to do with the quality of service provided, but by the expectations of others and the success, or otherwise, of operating within cash limits. The independent source of income necessary to maintain professional disinterest can no longer be assured.

Harrison and Pollitt (1994) have provided a useful framework for examining the process of change through their study of attempts to control professionals within the Health Service. Using their model it is possible to identify a number of phases in the changes wrought within the personal social services. Initial attention was given to cost savings and management by objectives and budgetary controls. This was followed by a focus on control over the processes and outcomes of service through the introduction of quality control and quality assurance measures. These were followed by management formulated statements of occupational competence, in which professional judgement and discretion was redefined as a technical process.

Directors of Social Services are now drawn into the corporate group of officers managing the affairs of the local authority. With the advent of information technology, administration is now dispersed. Each member of staff has access to the flow of information and the procedures intended to guide their actions.

The credibility of a social science-based education as the vehicle for qualifying training is undermined by a number of developments which have seen a shift of control over the professional qualifying process from the academy to employers. CCETSW itself has played a significant part in this process.

The move to the assessment of competence in the workplace against published standards had already cast doubts on the value to employers of time-served qualifying courses which relied on the evaluation of learning rather than performance outcomes. The possibility of accrediting prior learning and experience increased the doubts about the survival of taught courses that take a cohort of students through a cohesive programme of specific duration. A number of Social Service Departments have moved their training resources into the competence-assessed National Vocational Qualifications.

Social action has been reinstated into social work training within the last five years with the new Diploma in Social Work. The new qualification was driven by the demand from CCETSW for radical changes in practice and policies to address the disadvantage experienced as a result of discrimination, especially discrimination on the grounds of race. It was expected that the new generation of social workers would challenge the social-work agencies and the structures in which they operated. Conflict with the government was inevitable, and university-based social-work training has now come under further threat.

The recent history of social work, and that of its liberal professional intellectual mentors, is one of constant attrition and loss of credibility. Social workers are now required to justify their privileged position in terms of radical agendas set by others.

SOCIAL WORK IN THE 'POSTMODERN' AGE

There are a number of features in the present situation which indicate that social work as a professional activity may yet survive the political, social and economic onslaught on its credibility.

There is a growing awareness that competence is not readily assessed by performance alone. The judgements of professionally qualified social workers and managers are subject to scrutiny in the course of court proceedings and inquiries. The need for continual update on current practice and the ability to justify actions in terms of research and experience in a public arena is a significant one. The drive for this comes from the legal and quasi-legal authorities outside government. It also comes from the threat of litigation from failure to meet standards within service agreements or through appeal procedures. The quality of agreements themselves will be subject to monitoring within the quality-assurance processes. Social workers and others undertaking formal assessments will therefore need to have the skills, knowledge and understanding to determine not only what is appropriate but also to identify any impediments that might inhibit the effective use of the service provided. The choice must be an informed one and this may require careful exploration. The stakeholders of the service include not only clients serviced by their own 'professional' representatives, but also institutions such as the judiciary. Social workers may well be able to forge alliances that meet both service-user needs and professional ends. It is possible to identify the development of a specialist and highly professional social-work-based service, including service users. The traditional 'befriending' role is likely to return to in-house trained staff or to the ranks of volunteers.

The engagement of professionals in the orderly governance of the country will continue. The elaborate network of consultative groups at national level provides a shadow administration that undertakes much of the work on behalf of government in return for the opportunity to influence policy and regulations. In particular, the views of those likely to be charged with enacting legislation are important. Any legislation that proves unworkable and counter-productive will be discredited and become politically damaging to government. Ministers may also be reluctant to be seen to be de-professionalising particular services, such as child protection and community mental health, and to exposing themselves to the failure to protect the public. Social work presents a buffer between public criticism and ministerial responsibility. At organisational level, managers who have little insight into social-work practice will not be able to manage qualitative aspects of the service and may not wish to manage or take responsibility for others, thereby rationing services. Professionals are likely therefore to remain responsible for significant areas of work. The gravest danger to the status of the professional intellectuals lies not from ministers, who come and go, but from the possibility of corruption of the professional ideal by those amongst their ranks who distort their judgements in return for personal advantage.

The reining-in of public expenditure has provided the impetus for some practitioners to move out of the statutory provision into the independent sector. Experience in the United States suggests that a move towards longer-term partnerships between purchasers and providers is inevitable. The requirement of a knowledge of the social sciences will be supplemented, and not substituted, by the necessity to acquire a knowledge base in management and financial manage-ment. Quality assessment of need and provision will remain, al-though sharply focused in terms of a particular market niche.

Managers are not a single entity, and will need to cooperate with

their qualified staff when making decisions related to the achievement of professional goals. The social worker will remain the broker
between the various parties to an ever widening range of agreements
in the social-care field. They will also act as entrepreneurs in
widening the possibilities available to those parties.

The changes in training can be viewed as either a disintegration
of traditional routes to qualification or the integration of social-work
skills, knowledge and values into an increasingly diverse range of
occupations and activities. The expansion of counselling at the time
of retraction of social-work training in universities may be no more
than part of a process that will inevitably lead to further attention
beyond the plight of individuals to the circumstances of their lives.
As counsellors, volunteers, community nurses and others recognise
the need to address the social and material circumstances of their
clients' lives, so they will rediscover the influence of inter-personal
relationships on behaviour and attitudes. Thus the wheel turns full
circle, and each time the understanding of the social problems and
dilemmas is further enriched.

Professional social work comes at a price which will be costed
against that of other professionals and staff trained in-house operating within the same field. Social workers will therefore have to
demonstrate the advantages of their particular knowledge, understanding and skills. The demand for a broad-based knowledge of
social sciences, and the skills and experience required to apply it to
the resolution of social problems and dilemmas, will be a specialist
one. Training within the universities may therefore be confined to
postgraduate work, with a view to its application in specialist fields,
or in ways that will inform the management of social welfare
provision.

CONCLUSION

This chapter is an attempt to demonstrate the relationship between
the liberal members of the professional intellectual classes and the
evolution of modern social work. Their faith in the application of
social science to resolve social problems fuelled the development of
modern social work and shaped it within the context of an expanding
welfare state. The subsequent challenge to the achievements of the
welfare state by the radical left and then the radical right reflected a
growing recognition of the limitations of the modern approach to
social welfare in times of rapid economic and social change.

Initially, social work was little more than a feature of the administration of welfare. The professionalisation of social work came with recognition of the central importance of the relationship between worker and client and the contribution of psychology and sociology to the influences on inter-personal relationships. At all times the mentors of social work in academia, politics and the civil service were influencing developments. The cooperation between the mentors and the leaders of the professions was reinforced by a series of interlocking relationships.

The discrediting of social work is seen as part of the process of discrediting its mentors by those who seek to remould the present structure of the state by undermining the authority of those who maintain its services. Their radical influence is greatest when the processes and institutions through which orderly governance is maintained are strained. In response to the challenges posed, social-work education moves beyond the concern for personal experience and circumstances to reflect the new language, be it of social action or market economy. In this way social work is doing no more than following the drift of the mentors in adapting to their environment.

Whilst the present circumstances may indicate the demise of social work, there is evidence to suggest both that social work will survive at a more specialised and sophisticated level and that the significance of inter-personal relationships in human affairs is now more widely recognised than before.

Chapter 3

After social work?

John Clarke

Any consideration of the contemporary state of social work has to confront the sheer pace, scale and scope of change in which social work is enmeshed: from new legislation to local government reorganisation or from changing patterns of poverty and need to organisational restructuring. While change may now be a 'fact of life' for social work, the more difficult problem is how to make sense of it. It is this problem that makes the intersection of social work, social change and social theory so salient, since it offers the prospect of constructing an analytic grasp on the causes and directions of change. Given the intensity of change in and around social work, it is not surprising that the social theories which seem to have most to offer are those concerned with global or epochal transitions – the analyses of postmodernism and post-Fordism, in particular. In their different ways, each of these announces change as the dominant feature of the present and each identifies decisive shifts in the ordering of economic, political and cultural life.

This chapter has two main purposes. The first is to express some reservations about these 'posts' and to question whether their approaches can be usefully applied to the study of social welfare and social work. The second is to explore – at a less ambitious theoretical level – some of the changes currently shaping the future of social work by focusing on the intersection between processes of welfare restructuring and the specific position of social work within the welfare state in Britain. In many ways, this is a rather less exciting endeavour than working with the epochal scenarios of the 'posts', but I hope instead to offer a more grounded and more complex grasp of the social forces at work in and on social work.

THE STARTING POST: THE RISK OF HISTORICAL AMNESIA

I should begin with a confession. After the deluge of contemporary theorising which references its claim to novelty by defining itself by the prefix 'post', I have distinct problems with 'post' anything – whether it be postmodernism, post-Fordism, post-structuralism, post-feminism or any of the others. This unease rests primarily on an objection to a binary definition of history which subjects complicated problems of continuity and change to a simplifying juxtaposition of before and after. In the process, the past (that which is pre-the post-) is recurrently oversimplified, mystified and dismissed as no longer of interest. In the process, an apocalyptic transition to the new is effected. In what follows then, I am as concerned with how post-Fordism and postmodernism construct the past (Fordism and modernism) as with their analyses of the present and future. This may seem perverse, but I want to argue that we need a sense of our historical trajectories in order adequately to understand the present.

Post-Fordist – after the mass?

Ideas of post-Fordist patterns of industrial organisation address processes of economic reorganisation in the advanced industrial societies (in some versions these are capitalist economies) and identify movements towards flexibility and diversity. All varieties identify a Fordist past in which mass production and mass consumption meet in the monolithic economic and cultural architecture of the assembly line. Fordism is (narrowly) identified as a *system of production* which combines Taylorism (the fragmentation, specialisation and deskilling of labour) with mechanised/automated coordination and standardisation of production (involving what Marx called the real, as opposed to the formal, subsumption of labour – or the intensive exploitation of labour power as opposed to its extensive exploitation). The systemic organisation of mass production is linked to a *systemic organisation of mass consumption* through the creation of a mass market, supported by the high-wage economy. The development and coordination of mass consumption was an essential corollary of Fordist production as a guarantee that the potential profitability of the expanded range of commodities being produced would be realised.

Some versions (for example, Aglietta, 1979) have a more

expansive definition of Fordism as a '*regime of accumulation*'. Such analyses have treated the economic, social and political conditions of accumulation as systemic, linking the nexus of production and consumption to the role of the expanded state. The state took on an enhanced role in sustaining the appropriate conditions for capital accumulation through the management of relations between capital and labour, the management of macro-economic conditions and the coordination (nationally and internationally) of markets. The transition from Fordism to post-Fordism is seen as a consequence of (variously) the rise of differentiated markets; the availability of new technologies allowing production and product flexibility; the crisis of profitability in the late 1970s, and the intractability of labour in Fordism. Post-Fordism has become central to debates on restructuring – stressing the rise of 'flexible specialisation' as a link between production systems, new forms of labour use, differentiated consumption patterns and changes in the state.

I want to raise some doubts about the representation of the past in such accounts. The first doubt concerns the extent of Fordism and Fordist regimes in the context of capitalist economies which remained resolutely 'pre-Fordist' – that is those that continued to seek profitability through the extensive exploitation of labour power or which were just catching up with Taylorism (Hudson, 1988; Sayer and Walker, 1992, ch. 5). That is, if we take the regimes model from Aglietta we have to confront societies which involved ill-fitting combined regimes and where the conditions of success for some forms of capital are not those of others. For example, there have been vigorous arguments about whether Britain ever achieved 'full Fordism' (Cochrane, 1989; Hudson, 1988).

Second, I think it is important to point to ways in which the use of the concept of mass consumption relies on an over-exaggeration of massification against evidence of diversity. We need to pay some attention to the *limited access* to mass consumption outside of core sectors of labour (those positioned inside the high-wage economy), since participation in mass consumption was itself cash-limited, and to remember the ways in which much apparently mass consumption consumed not the products of Fordism but of pre-Fordist sweated trades (such as clothing). We also need not to forget earlier arguments about the way mass consumption (and especially mass culture) intersected with forms of cultural differentiation based on *status terms*: the constant reworking of taste/privilege as aspirational structures, not merely a high versus mass culture binary distinction.

Holidays, for example, have been the site of continuous struggles to reconstitute varieties of difference and exclusivity against 'mass' (that is, proletarian) access through shifting sites and forms of leisure activities (Clarke and Critcher, 1984).

More abstractly, there are also issues about the existence of forms of *hidden differentiation* which are concealed by equating mass distribution with mass consumption. I have argued elsewhere about the importance of sustaining a distinction between the moment of exchange and the moment of consumption in the analysis of consumer cultures (Clarke, 1991: ch. 4). Consumption needs to be analytically distinguished from the processes of distribution and exchange if we are to understand it as a field of social and cultural practices which take place in differentiated settings. Much consumption as a social practice is 'private', concealing transformative labours of 'customisation' – the creation and extraction of use values – and the gendered distribution of those labours. As a consequence, I think this means that the concept of a Fordist regime is unthinkable without the family/home as a central articulatory site through which the social relationships of production and consumption are connected through a particular gendered division of labour.

Turning to the most expansive conception of Fordism (as a regime of accumulation), the idea of a *Fordist state* raises major problems of comparative diversity in the varieties of forms taken by the expanded state and in the very different periodisations which are visible. Thus, Esping-Anderson's work on different welfare regimes identifies different varieties of the expanded state (social democratic, corporatist and residual), all of which obtained in countries which have been assumed to operate Fordist regimes. The assumed congruence of Fordism as a systemic structure of production, consumption and state form downgrades questions of political processes and the diversity of their outcomes in favour of economic or technological determinism. These issues suggest some problems which need to be addressed in analysing the present. First, there is a question about the empirical extent of post-Fordism/flexible specialisation strategies and whether these should form the focus of attention as opposed to looking at an *expanded repertoire of strategies for capital accumulation* (for example, Hudson, 1988; Rustin, 1989; Sayer and Walker, 1992).

Second, there are questions about what a *post-Fordist state* would look like (Burrows and Loader, 1994). Are its major relations to a new regime of accumulation the processes of deregulation or privatisation? Is it that the state is more differentiated in its outputs or is it subject to a process of de-differentiation *vis-à-vis* the 'mixed economy'? Is there a 'recommodification' of the realm of public welfare? Are there more flexible patterns of post-bureaucratic organisation? All of these processes (and more) have been identified in recent developments in state forms and processes. At present, I think there is a substantial gap between generalisations about the nature of the state in post-Fordism (or in the transition to post-Fordism) and the empirical substance of welfare restructurings (Clarke, forthcoming). Equally importantly, the somewhat impoverished view of social relations in the Fordist model (dominated by class or 'productionist' understandings) lags somewhat behind the analysis of social welfare in terms of its articulations of class, 'race' and gender (Williams, 1994).

I think that there are two particular problems about the application of the Fordism/post-Fordism analysis to social welfare. The first concerns whether the organisations, labour processes and 'products' of the old welfare state can be meaningfully described as 'Fordist'. They do not appear to be Fordist in any direct sense: mass-production systems and processes were not forms of organising social welfare. Nor can an argument be sustained which draws an analogy between the systems of Fordist industrial production and the 'bureaucratic monoliths' of welfare provision. The labour processes and organisational forms of the welfare state were always more than bureaucratic, depending heavily on the exercise of different types of professional judgement and discretion. They produced welfare benefits and services which involved complex classificatory schemas of types of 'client', 'condition', 'need' and responses – rather than a 'mass' product.

The second problem concerns the emergent, rather than the past, forms of welfare organisation. Even if the old welfare state was not Fordist, it might still be argued that the restructurings of social welfare have produced post-Fordist tendencies: for example, in the creation of new service or organisational fragmentation; new forms of service differentiation or new flexibilities in the organisation and use of labour. While such trends are certainly visible (as in health and social care), it is more difficult to tell whether these are intrinsically or essentially post-Fordist developments. Some of these changes involve efforts to establish older forms of labour discipline (Taylorism) on labour forces whose autonomy has proved resistant to managerial control (for example, Pollitt, 1990; Rustin, 1994).

These changes go on alongside efforts to create flexible labour forces, new human resource management approaches or decentralised systems (Flynn, 1994). The direction of change is not unilinear but involves an expanded range of strategies for organising and controlling welfare processes. The problem with the post-Fordist argument is that it too readily assumes that every 'flexibility' or 'fragmentation' is an expression of the essential principles of post-Fordist development. By contrast, I think it is necessary to explore how – through what complex of processes and forces – the organisation of welfare has come to reflect (or mimic) some features of contemporary business organisation. The later sections of this chapter return to these issues, but first there is a detour via the other 'post' – postmodernism.

Postmodernism – the end of civilisation as we know it?

The problem with the postmodernist story which stresses a cultural transition from monolithic to diverse is that there is an even greater diversity of specifications about what the postmodern might be – for example, greater diversity; the proliferation of difference; de-differentiation; indifference; the plural, contradictory, fragmented subject; new communicative technologies; the aestheticisation of everyday life; the hyperreal; the loss of aura/authority/authenticity; the collapse of the master narratives or even Baudrillard's proposition that 'reality flickers'. Versions of these contemporary characteristics are juxtaposed against a past which is variously defined as hierarchic, hieratic, mass, based in unitary subjects, embodying authorial and authoritative cultural and theoretical production and which is monolithic, if not totalitarian, in its cultural forms.

Again, I have some problems with the past as it is told in postmodernist tales. I find it difficult to recognise a past which features either (1) no differences or (2) simple/binary/hierarchic differences. These repress the evidence of exceedingly complex patterns of cultural differentiation around class (and its complex subdivisions); the complex intersection of class and ethnicity (especially in the United States) and gender (the diverse particular formations of patriarchy); the complex cultural architecture in which identities based in and created through community, locality, region, nation, religion, or 'taste cultures' (which are not solely the terrain of patrician versus plebeian taste, or high versus popular culture). In a different way, it may also be worth noting the explosion of subject positionings discerned by Foucauldian researchers which begin in the nineteenth century – in the bio/psycho complexes' architecture of 'race', gender, sexuality, ability and age. The richness of these discursive classifications suggests the availability of a wide range of differentiated and complex subject positions.

This leads to a different question about the postmodernist transition: what is *different about differences*? I think it is possible to discern two versions of answers to this question. The first is that postmodernism is the cultural effect of the *politicisation of difference* (the enunciation of differences which have not hitherto been represented) as new collective subjects form themselves through their differentiation and against their absence (Williams, 1992 and 1994). If that is so, there is an act of forgetting which goes on in many (though not all) claims to theorising postmodernism, which is to appropriate the 'diversity effect' in the symbolic realm of these representational struggles and detach them from their social and political bases. There is also, I fear, a further historical objection that many of these struggles (and others) have gone on prior to their eruption in the postmodern but are historically unregarded (particularly those around the cultural politics of 'race', gender and sexuality).

Despite these reservations, this view of the politicisation of differences seems more compelling than the more agnostic varieties of postmodernism, which have treated the proliferation of differences as overshadowed by *an indifference to differences*. Here, all differences are equally valorised and valueless, since none is (or can claim to be) authentic or significant. This 'wild pluralism' has its undoubted attractions, not least in the way it underpins the postmodern repertoire of irony, playfulness, detachment and cynicism. But it is also intimately bound up with the de-politicising agnosticism of postmodernism which has enraged many critics. While sharing this sense of frustration, I think that there remain other problems buried in postmodernist bifurcations of past and present (see also Clarke, 1991: ch. 2).

I have some difficulty with accounts of the historical past which treat it as a field of authoritative cultural practice or characterised by the dominance of 'master narratives'. I have trouble matching this account of history with those histories in which people were constantly *'in trouble with the authorities'*. More specifically, I mistrust the representation of the past as a time when authorities were successfully exercised (that is, when the master narratives told stories that people believed). To erect this version of history, you have to forget all the other stories – the Utopians, the primitive rebels, the prefiguratives and the radicals (and in some cases the conservatives, though it seems that their stories always come back to haunt us). You also have to forget that cynicism and scepticism are not our invention – that even those who did not tell *other* stories cannot simply be read (with the vast condescension of hindsight) as 'believers'. This variety of historical amnesia reproduces the most mundane functionalist error about history – which is that the winners get to tell the tale and it is their stories which survive. I am not denying that they did win and that their victories are significant, but I am not willing to do so at the expense of suppressing resistances (that, after all, is how the winners won).

These issues about authority have particular salience for the study of social work. It is tempting to read its recent history as exemplifying the transition from modernism to postmodernism through tracing the impact of social and cultural diversity on its field of practice. Both the proliferation of 'differences' and their politicisation would seem to confirm the postmodern perspective – as would the challenges which they represent to social work's claims to legitimate authority. Nevertheless, there is a danger here of projecting a past in which social work was authoritative and received deferentially or acquiescently by those subjected to it. But this will not do. Social work's past is marked by challenges, resistances and refusals in both collective and individual forms. From its nineteenth-century origins, social work has been viewed ambiguously and sceptically by both its beneficiaries and commentators on it (see, *inter alia*, Fido, 1977; Gordon, 1992; and Hobson, 1896)

After the post?

Both postmodernism and post-Fordism have exerted a considerable influence in reshaping social theory, giving a central place to social change in the process. My unease about them, though, centres on the ways in which they construct the past against which the new is defined. Both are subject to 'historical amnesia', and there are dangers attached to taking them up and applying them – as if they were unproblematic – to the study of social welfare and social work. Before moving on, I want to suggest that what these perspectives have to offer needs to be viewed ambiguously. Both, I think, manage to convey a sense of the pace and scale of change, even though they neglect problems of continuity and the persistence of the old in the new. Second, they draw attention to social conditions, relations and processes as multiple, diverse rather than unidimensional, even though they make the past monolithic. Third, they point to the salience of new or emergent economic, political, cultural and organisational strategies, even though they underestimate the persistence of older forms. Fourth, they point to ways in which previously would-be authoritative positions have been destabilised, although they overestimate their past authority.

These observations are intended to suggest that my problems with the 'posts' are not about whether 'something is going on', but that the ways in which changes are being appropriated theoretically are flawed. I am concerned by the way in which the posts manage to both conflate and flatten difference (even while celebrating it). In the process I want to remember some of the things that are currently the subject of 'historical amnesia' – to hold on to a past which was less monolithic than its presentation implies and to resist the implication that we have moved unproblematically to a new order. At the same time, I want to develop an approach to the present and future of social work which sees these processes of transformation as more partial, more uneven, more contradictory and less finished than viewing them from the vantage point of the posts would imply. To do so means dealing with the particular social processes and forces which are transforming social work rather than assuming that social work may simply exemplify the big issues identified in the posts.

MARKETS, MIXED ECONOMIES, MOTHERS AND MANAGERS – THE RESTRUCTURING OF WELFARE

In developing these concerns, I want to focus on the recent and continuing processes of welfare restructuring. Although these involve both global and national economic and social changes, these contexts are mediated through specific political and cultural processes, which in Britain places the neo-Conservative politics of welfare at the centre of restructuring. Those politics have included the constant demand for constraint and reductions in public spending (particularly on welfare) and a generalised hostility towards state intervention. Nevertheless, the fortunes of the welfare state – and social work within it – cannot simply be read off from neo-Conservative rhetoric about 'anti-statism', but involve more complex processes of restructuring. These have addressed the political, economic and organisational contexts in which social work has historically been located and in which its future is being constructed. In this context, I cannot do more than sketch arguments which have been developed more extensively elsewhere. In an effort to simplify these arguments, I have tried to identify four main strands.

The first concerns the processes of *marketisation* in relation to social welfare. This I take to refer to two related phenomena – the sponsored development of competition in the provision of welfare services and the introduction of 'internal markets' within public service organisations as a way of making them mimic market relationships (see, *inter alia*, Taylor-Gooby and Lawson, 1993; Le Grand and Bartlett, 1993). This has also been described as the creation of the 'contracting state' (Harden, 1992), which may be understood as referring to both senses of the word 'contracting'. It conveys the move towards contractual modes of relationship as a central feature of the organisation of service provision as well as the reduction of direct service provision by public institutions. Le Grand's development of the idea of 'quasi-markets' is an important one in identifying the artificial, imitative and regulated nature of these marketised relationships and is reflected in the distinct – and peculiar – position of the 'customer' in such markets (see also Clarke, 1994).

Such market-making processes are linked to the development of *mixed economies of welfare*. I have a preference for referring to these in the plural, rather than the conventional singular usage for social policy for the simple reason that there is not a single mixed economy. There are multiple mixed economies – with variations for different aspects of welfare and local rather than national formations of mixed economies (Charlesworth, *et al.*, 1994a). That is, there are sectorally and spatially differentiated mixed economies. Although it is important to be careful about not adopting the neo-Conservative view of the past as one dominated by public welfare 'monopolies' (and recognising that there have always been mixed economies of welfare), what is clear is that there has been a sustained attempt to shift the balance of provision towards the independent sector of private and voluntary providers (Langan and Clarke, 1993). In the process, direct provision through what we used to refer to as the welfare state has been decentred and dislocated to a substantial extent. These processes have had the effect of blurring the boundaries between state and non-state welfare provision, since they may be seen as contracting-*out* activities previously performed by state agencies but may also be seen as bringing independent agencies *into* new relationships of partnership with, regulation by, and even dependence on the state (Charlesworth *et al.*, 1994b).

Third, there is the continuing transfer of responsibilities from *formal to informal provision* – towards 'care by the community'. Although this is most explicit in the field of social care, this is only part of a wider privatisation of welfare responsibilities, including aspects of health, education, income maintenance for adolescents and parental responsibilities for criminal behaviour. The processes of familialisation have been extensively discussed in social policy and their specifically gendered character have received much attention, so I do not intend to pursue them here. What I do want to draw attention to is one particular element in this redrawing of the public–private boundary, which tends to be hidden in the concentration on what is being 'devolved' to the family. These shifts are double edged, since they also create new forms of discipline and surveillance over family life: whether this is the criminalisation of parents, the Child Support Agency's interventions or the assessment of carers in the preparation of community care packages. Here, too, the boundaries between public and private are being blurred as the state both transfers tasks and responsibilities to the familial realm while simultaneously extending the scope of surveillance and regulation of that realm. For example, the expansion of forms of voluntary and informal care, sometimes linked to 'payment for caring' (Ungerson, 1993), opens up new issues about how such caring work is to be organised and supervised – or made subject to labour discipline.

Finally, I want to draw attention to processes of *managerialisation*. I shall spend rather more time on these, since they have proved less visible in social policy analysis than the other strands and they have profound consequences for the world of social work. In talking about managerialisation, I am concerned with two related phenomena: first, the nature of modes of organisational coordination (the principles on which organisations are organised and interorganisational relationships are constructed); and second the nature of organisational regimes (the characteristic patterns of structures, cultures and power within organisations).

We may approach the first of these via two rather banal observations. One is that all organisations require coordination and thus what distinguishes them are their predominant principles of coordination. The second, more specific, point is that neither markets nor mixed economies run themselves: they require *agents* to make them work.

In the contemporary public sector the preferred form of that agency is management. More particularly, it is management as opposed to administrative bureaucracy or professionalism. The transformations of welfare involving markets and mixed economies seem naturally to require managers as the embodiment of the types of skills, knowledges and capacities (above all the capacity to 'do the right thing') needed to make such processes work efficiently (du Gay, forthcoming; Newman and Clarke, 1994).

Behind this banal starting point is a more complex issue about why managerialism is the preferred mode of organisational coordination. Condensed in this revival of managerialism are a number of economic, political and ideological transitions (see Clarke and Newman, 1993a). These include the wider setting of the reconstruction of managerial power in the 1980s – under the banner of the 'right to manage' – which involved the sustained destruction of extra- and intra-organisational inhibitions to the exercise of managerial discretion. These processes included the reduction of trade-union rights and powers and the extension of managerial control over how to use labour forces. Although pioneered in industrial settings, such developments have also been visible in public services (for example, in the impact of compulsory competitive tendering). A rather different dimension involves the reworking of the ideology of managerialism itself – or, more accurately, the discourses of different managerialisms which link the broader ideology to variants of how management is to be practised (and to what being a manager means). Most visible in this reworking has been the 'Excellence' discourse associated with Tom Peters – propounding a more dynamic, visionary, customer-centred version of managerial leadership (Clarke and Newman, 1993a; Woods, 1989). Thirdly, there are important political articulations between the generalised revival of managerialism and the definition of the crisis of the welfare state which have underpinned the installation of the managerial mode of coordination in the reconstruction of welfare (Clarke, et al., 1994).

In this last point it is possible to see the links between modes of coordination and organisational regimes. Although there are multiple dimensions to, and definitions of, the crisis of the welfare state, the neo-Conservative attack on welfare has consistently linked the generalised fiscal crisis of welfare to a more specific critique of the organisational patterns of welfare provision associated with the social democratic consensus. This has included attacks on 'provider power': its bureaucratic rigidities, inflexibility, professional imperialism, insensitivity to users, impermeability to the dynamics of competition as well as the intrusive 'dogma' of political interference and control (particularly within the welfare systems of the local state). Although this has provided the foundation for both marketisation and changing the balance of mixed economies, it has also supported the introduction of managerial modes of coordination into public-sector bodies as the precondition of reshaping their organisational regimes.

We have argued this in more detail elsewhere (Clarke and Newman, 1993b; Newman and Clarke, 1994), but I want to make a couple of major points about these processes. The characteristic organisational regime of the social democratic welfare state was one of professional bureaucracy (or bureau-professionalism) in which the dominant modes of coordination were those of rational administration and professional discretion. Both modes embodied the Fabian model of social welfare – the application of expertise to the solution of social problems. Both involved laying claim to specific sorts of power; both constructed specific modes of coordination (hierarchical authority and collegial relations); both involved specific sorts of relationships with users and potential users of welfare services; and both laid claim to distinctive forms of neutrality (bureaucratic rationality and professional knowledge and values). The articulation of these modes of coordination in the organisational regimes of the welfare state underpinned its characteristic organisational structures and cultures, its characteristic disputes and conflicts, its characteristic patterns of dealing with 'citizens' and 'clients', and conditioned its uneven articulations with local forms of political representation. This regime also underpinned the impenetrability of specific domains of welfare practice (medical discretion, the curriculum and so on) to direct control by central government.

The collapse of the *ancien régime* is not solely the effect of neo-Conservatism. Such bureau-professional regimes of welfare faced an astonishingly diverse range of critiques – from varieties of left and liberal democratic positions, from feminists, from minority ethnic groups, and from alliances mobilising or speaking for service users as well as from the Institute of Economic Affairs (IEA) and other think tanks of the right (Clarke, 1993a). The significance of the neo-Conservative attack is two-fold. First, and most mundanely, they got themselves into the position to do something about it. Second, they articulated diverse critiques into a relatively systematic version which aimed to speak for the people against the state or, more precisely, for the welfare 'customer' against the 'provider power' embodied in the old regime (Clarke, 1994).

IN WHAT STATE? THE CONDITION OF SOCIAL WORK

All of this brings me (at last) to the issue of social work. It is tempting to suggest that diagnoses of the present condition of social work reflect the diversity of perceptions of the wider state of welfare. At the extremes, these range from the view that the welfare state has done remarkably well to survive the onslaughts of the 1980s (Hills, 1990) to the more pessimistic scenarios of crisis, dismemberment and collapse (Krieger, 1987). Nevertheless, I do not think this will do. Such equivalences are not sufficiently attentive to the peculiarities of social work and its particular trajectory through the welfare state. As the would-be 'fifth social service', social work was late arriving in the welfare state. It was strangely positioned – at the heart of the local rather than national state. It was also strangely constituted – in the post-Seebohm figure of the generic social worker. And, of course, it was the victim of 'bad timing' – in crisis almost from the point of its creation (Langan, 1993a). Despite all these peculiarities, however, we might note that its regime was classically one of bureau-professionalism, even if the professional side of this combination was always relatively fragile.

It is equally tempting to identify social work with the tendencies to fragmentation identified in both post-Fordism and postmodernism. From such a starting point, one could point to the fragmentation of different specialisms, the different tendencies inscribed in the legislation affecting children and community care, the pressures to be attentive to difference and diversity driven from below by 'client' pressures and from above by 'customer-centredness', and the organisational fragmentations both within social services departments (decentralisation, purchaser-provider splits and so on) and beyond them in the multiplication of care providers. While I think all of these tendencies are significant, I am concerned about the application of the monolith/fragmentation argument to them, since it presumes a past in which there was *a* social work.

It will come as no surprise to find that I am rather sceptical about such a unified conception. I think it is more productive to think of social work as always/already fragmentary from its nineteenth-century origins and to see its history as repeatedly marked by tensions between fragmentation and integration, in which a variety of strategies have been used to try to construct a coherence or unity out of the fragments (Clarke, 1993b). At different times, one might look to the casework method, the psychological sciences, the idea of social work itself, generic social work or the systems approach as providing the bases for more or less successful attempts at integration. As a result, the current tendencies towards fragmentation need to be specified more precisely, both in terms of this being one of many fragmentations in social work's history and in terms of what it is that is being fragmented (for example, is it the practice of social work or its organisational forms?).

I think it is worth treating the last decade or so of social work's history in terms of the way in which it has been traversed – or perhaps worked over – by a variety of social forces, rather than trying to identify one or two dominant tendencies. This way of viewing the contemporary state of social work makes it possible to identify the contradictory impulses and pressures to which social work has been subjected rather than establishing linear directions. What follows is necessarily sketchy, but I think that each of the forces identified has contributed distinctively to the crisis of social work and to the forms in which that crisis is being resolved.

Since social work has been above all a service directed at the poor, the starting point must be the impact of the changing shape of poverty itself – both in quantitative and qualitative terms. The deepening of material inequalities through the 1980s is the 'dark side' of all the drama and excitement of welfare restructuring. In this deepening, we can see the combined effects of market inequalities, the effects of a tax and fiscal policy aimed at 'easing the tax burden' on individual and corporate wealth creators, and the move towards a more 'lean and mean' approach to public services and benefits. Cumulatively, there are more poor people and they have become relatively poorer in respect of the overall distribution of income. Both the direct and secondary effects of poverty have consequences for social work in the form of client bombardment. More particularly, the shifting embodiments of inequality have specific types of salience for social work: for example, in the 'feminisation' and 'racialisation' of poverty and in the intersection of disability and poverty (Cochrane, 1993a; Oppenheim, 1993).

There is a second demand-side process that has had significant impact on social work, which might be described as 'representational' struggles. Social work has been a particularly clear focal point for cultural politics and equality campaigns from a range of sources, focused on gender, sexuality, disability, age and ethnicity (Taylor, 1993). Some of these are about the representation of need; some about the distribution of power between professionals, users and carers; some about the relationship between social work and the family; some about rights and some about representation within the social-work profession itself. These have made their mark on social work and have, to a limited extent, been internalised in the commitment to and language of 'anti-oppressive practice'. This is not the place to explore the issues which these struggles have raised in any detail, but it is important to note how these processes of cultural and political struggle around identity, rights and representation have constituted 'difference', 'diversity' and 'fragmentation' in very specific ways in the context of social work. They are also one focus of contradictory pressures in relation to government policies – manifested on the one hand in moves towards greater sensitivity to individual circumstances (in the community care and children's legislation), and on the other, in the hostility to 'ologies and isms' (a recurrence of the longer-running 'bad theories versus common sense' argument).

Such pressures have also intersected with the greater public visibility of social work, particularly around work with children and families, to create a crisis of direction (Franklin and Parton, 1991). The 'damned if we do, damned if we don't' double bind of social work intervention in relation to child abuse has been extensively discussed – its significance here is the way in which it has multiplied the different sorts of pressure bearing on social work – enquiries, inspections, media reportage, varieties of guidance and so on. These pressures are now being reproduced in community care in such issues as elder abuse, the 'dangerousness' of mentally ill people and so on. These multiplying pressures take place in the wider context of the fiscal crisis of the state (O'Connor, 1973). I do not propose to take too long on this subject either, but there are three salient points. First, the crisis has been constructed, discursively, as a fiscal one. Crises are not naturally occurring phenomena, but have to be made to *mean* something. In the last twenty years, the overarching meaning has been articulated around the Public Sector Borrowing Requirement (PSBR). Second, public spending has predominantly been made to mean public spending on welfare. Third, the crisis of the welfare state is, in large part, about the crisis of relations between different welfare states – central and local (Cochrane, 1993b). This is a relatively terse way of getting to the point that the context of crisis is not simply out there as a backdrop to social work's fortunes, but that social work is intimately linked to the fiscal, political, governmental and organisational forms in which that crisis has been taking shape.

Finally, it is important to note some of the more professional and organisational tendencies that are currently present in the reconstruction of social work. On the one hand, we have the divergent models for social work embedded in the major pieces of legislation affecting its function. Where the Children Act emphasises partnership, juridification and 'super-professionalism' (the latter two particularly in the field of child protection), the NHS and Community Care Act residualises social work as one form of provision amongst many in the care market, to be purchased by care managers who need not be social workers (Langan, 1993b; Langan and Clarke, 1994). These divergent tendencies undercut lingering notions of genericism and introduce new organisational divisions into the world of the social services department. At the same time, social work is having its own encounter with the emergence of the new public-sector management – the processes of managerialisation (Kelly, 1991; Langan and Clarke, 1994). The case for social work needing new and better management is both familiar (in the common elements that it shares with the rest of the public sector) and distinctive (in the specific formulations of strategic and devolved management capacities and systems that are needed).

What is important here is the way managerialisation is both related to other tendencies (the political initiatives of neo-Conservatism; the three E's of the fiscal crisis, the legislation of community care) and is an independent agent in its own right – embedded in management education and development, private- and public-sector management writing and the roles of agencies such as the Audit Commission, the Office for Public Management and the Local Government Management Board as well as the initiatives of specific local authorities. Organisational and managerial reform, reconstruction and re-engineering have become a focal concern, manifesting themselves in restructurings, cultural change programmes, devolved and decentralised systems, performance management and the rest.

To pull all this together, it is worth returning to Gramsci's distinction between the 'organic' and 'conjunctural' features of a crisis. The organic – or deep-rooted – elements of the contemporary crisis of social work can be discerned in three particular configurations. The first may be defined as the inherent contradictions or instabilities of the social democratic form of the welfare state (its economic, fiscal and political settlements). The second may be defined as the instability of the social settlement of social democracy: its limited universalism rooted in the normative model of the heterosexual, patriarchal and ethnicised family (Williams, 1993). The third may be identified as the contradictory and unstable nature of the bureau-professional regimes of the welfare state and of the specific form of that regime in social work. In distinguishing these configurations as organic, I am trying to draw attention to the ways in which the place of social work in the welfare state meant that it was subject, from its creation, to contradictions and potential instabilities. Each of these organic features, however, takes a conjunctural form – the specific way in which those tensions are manifested and worked on in their intersection with other elements that make up the particular form of crisis currently being experienced. The present conjuncture is one in which the multiple forces at work on social work have been articulated with neo-Conservative agendas for restructuring welfare – and social work's place within it.

I want to argue that the specific form that the crisis has taken is a crisis of the 'regime' – the crisis of bureaucracy and professionalism which have become untenable positions both independently and in their combination as an organisational regime. This, although it creates an uncomfortable mouthful, should more properly be described as a crisis of the 'political-bureau-professional regime', since the regime involved an articulated complex of multiple modes of coordination: local political representation, bureaucratic administration and professional judgement. Each of these modes has been undercut and challenged by the changes of the 1980s and 1990s. Local political representation has been marginalised by the shift of public resources to non-elected agencies and quangos, while being more tightly circumscribed in what remains in local government by expanded central government control of both policy and resources. Bureaucratic administration has been challenged by the promise of a more dynamic and entrepreneurial approach to managing organizations. Professionalism has been placed on the defensive by the assertion of customer-centred models of provision, the fragmentations of professional tasks and the expectation that professionals can be disciplined by the creation of devolved managerial systems and new responsibilities for resource control. This shifting field of organisational power has both created the space for management as

a new force and its development is intimately linked to the expansion
of managerial authority.

AFTER SOCIAL WORK?

When I was asked to provide a title for this chapter, the phrase 'after
social work' came immediately to mind. It sounds rather apocalyptic,
it is true, but in this section I want to give it some substance, even
though it is essentially speculative. The forms in which the crisis of
social work is being resolved – the dominant tendencies that can be
discerned – are ones which will make it increasingly impossible to
refer to something called social work with any degree of confidence.
Social work is once again being subject to processes of fragmentation or disintegration, and it is less clear whether there are any
countervailing re-integrative tendencies or focal points which are as
powerful. These disintegrative tendencies have both organisational
and professional forms (although the two are, of course, inter-
connected). What follows is a brief list of these tendencies: some of
them can already be seen in social work, while others are visible
elsewhere in local government or the wider world of public services,
but have potential implications for social work.

The first is the rise of the 'arm's length' or 'agency' model of
service governance, exemplified most clearly in the Next Steps
initiatives in the Civil Service (Ditch, 1993; Ling, 1994). Such
changes involve downgrading patterns of political representation and
bureaucratic administration as modes of coordination and installing
a managerial mode instead (the Benefits Agency, NHS Management
Executive and so on). Such models also have an affinity with the
quango-based direction of public spending, dubbed the 'new magistracy' by John Stewart (1993a), in which non-elected and non-
accountable boards have taken on greater power over public services.
There is no reason to think that such models will not have increasing
significance for social work, not least because of the implications of
joint working with an increasingly managerialised Health Service.

Such joint working or partnership developments form the second
tendency, visible both in community care and child protection work.
Although taking different forms, both fields of social-work practice
raise the prospect of services being defined and delivered in the
interstices between organisations rather than within the existing
structural forms. Despite the lead agency role for Social Service
Departments in community care, for example, both strategies for,

and the practice of, community care are likely to move increasingly to the spaces between organisations. I do not mean to underestimate the importance of the structural tensions between organisations (of power, culture, professional agendas and the like) which have bedevilled inter-organisational working in the past, but the conditions under which organisational power can be sustained and defended have changed significantly.

Third, there is the increasing fragmentation of the world of the Social Service Department along a number of different axes – professional or service distinctions (for example, between child protection, child care and community care); organisational restructurings around the purchaser/provider split in community care (including the possible divestment of service provision to trust status or as independent trading units); and pressures towards increased devolution and decentralisation away from a strategic core. These tendencies have destabilised both the generic unity of social work and its familiar organisational proxy, the Social Services Department. They raise the questions of what social work is, and where it is practised. They point unerringly to the mixed economy of provision, with multiple agencies offering different types of social care services.

It is worth remarking that all of these tendencies have their reflections in the wisdom of the new managerialism. The first (the agency model) appears as the demand for managers to be granted 'the right to manage' without unnecessary political 'meddling'. The second (joint working) has its managerial surrogate in the concern for partnerships and synergy as the basis of 'value-added' management and in the managerial critique of the inward focus of traditional bureaucracies. The third cluster (fragmentation) is captured in the managerial concerns with 're-engineering' organisations, with establishing cost or profit centres, with developing a strategic core and with getting 'close to the customer'. Such parallels are not a coincidence, given that the managerial mode is the chosen agent of public-sector restructuring.

In Figure 3.1, I have tried to draw out a scenario for the future of social work in the form of an organisation chart c. 1999. It represents what might be the outcome of these tendencies if they persist in strong forms. I admit to some reservations about it. On the one hand, it does not fully capture the sense of 'cultural revolution' associated with the new managerialism since it is mainly focused on structures. As a consequence, it does not convey the sense of missions, quality assurance, corporate cultures, new working relationships and identities that are an essential part of the current managerialist transformations. Nor does it convey the changed working conditions and controls to which the employees would be subject. On the other hand, it is a deliberate overreading of the dominant tendencies. As it is properly subject to all sorts of qualifications about the outcome of different sorts of struggles (over the power and effect of service users, local politicians and professionals or between different sorts of 'cores' and their peripheries). It is not intended to convey a view that there is (or will be) a new welfare order which is free of conflict and contradiction. On the contrary, the new regimes both change and multiply the sites of instabilities and tensions (Clarke and Newman, forthcoming).

However, Figure 3.1 represents a projection of the future of social work based on the tendencies identified above. What I hope is striking about it is the fact that social work is to be found nowhere within it. Nobody – and no organisation – does social work. No one is employed as a social worker. It represents a future in which social work has been fragmented into different types of service (child protection; family services and community care) and where those services have been re-organised around the distinction between purchasers and providers. Not all of the services are organised through (much less provided by) local authorities – both child protection and community care have been moved to more independent positions within structures of multi-agency direction and control. Each 'agency' will have developed its own managerial structures (for personnel, finance, audit and so on) alongside its service role. The provider side is only lightly sketched in, but it will have become both more complex (as once public services are divested into trusts or floated off as businesses) and more organised as providers seek forms of combination ('consortia' in the figure) in order to organise contractual relationships with purchasers.

However, if this was the outcome, the big question is whether it would matter? It could be argued that such changes are merely organisational and that what we now talk of as social work will go on being practised in a number of different organisational settings and sites. This might even be a situation where social work returns to its fragmentary origins: a diversity of ways of working with those in need in a variety of contexts. Alternatively, it might be suggested that such changes are purely nominal – the practice of social work will go on even though the name may disappear. I confess that my

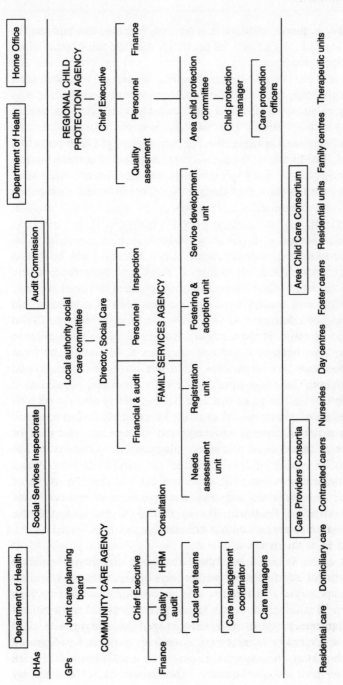

Figure 3.1 After social work, *c.* 1999?

own view is more pessimistic than this, because the current re-structurings and the principles on which they are based pose some very serious problems.

First, in a climate of continuing public spending constraint, such changes are likely to exacerbate tendencies towards social care being services which are residualised and focused on narrowing definitions of 'danger' and 'need'. This will increase the prospect of such services being seen as stigmatised and stigmatising. These processes are intensified by the shift towards organisational structures centred on autonomous (or semi-autonomous) 'business units', since such structures tend towards focusing on their 'core business' rather than more general public service objectives.

Second, although the creation of new organisational structures and managerial authority in public services have been legitimated by reference to their greater efficiency, they also create new costs and problems of coordination. Some of these are recognised in the growing literature on markets and quasi-markets in social welfare, such as issues of transaction costs and processes of regulation and monitoring of contracted service provision (for example, LeGrand and Bartlett, 1993; Hudson, 1994). But other issues have become visible in the 'boundary disputes' between NHS bodies and local authorities over the separation of health care and social care. Although both sides have articulated claims about how the patient's/customer's needs are to be met best, such disputes also reveal how boundaries and definitions of need are inextricably linked to structures of resource control and budgetary ownership. The idea of 'ownership' (whether of resources, missions or objectives) is supposed to be one of the strengths of the newly marketised and managerialised organisational structures but it is also the source of 'perverse incentives' for organisations to remove or reduce claims on their resources. Fragmentation, in its many forms, multiplies the number of inter-organisational boundaries and thus increases the potential for such disputes.

Third, a significant effect of these changes is to reshape the nature and conditions of 'discretion' within social work. In the old bureau-professional regime, discretion was a complex process in which professional judgement could be exercised within statutory and bureaucratic framings. In emergent managerialised regimes, professional judgement is increasingly bound up with, and potentially subordinated to, managerial imperatives concerning corporate objectives and resource control. The devolution of managerial responsibilities (particularly in relation to resources and budgets) is intended both to 'empower the front line' of organisations and to constrain professional autonomy by having professionals internalise budgetary disciplines. The result is that professional processes and categories of evaluation are compounded with managerial categories of cost, efficiency and risk. Such 'hybrid' calculations intensify pressures on those performing such roles and are, at best, unlikely to make for more 'transparent' representations of users' needs (Clarke, 1994). This process of integrating professional and managerial principles forms one variant of what Williams (1994) has called 'managed diversity', in which the demands for greater attention to social diversity in the provision of welfare services is taken account of but framed (and dominated) by organisational imperatives and criteria.

Finally, the dismemberment of social work generates a problem of identity, values and loyalties. While the old bureau-professional regime of the Social Services Department had characteristic tensions and contradictions, it nevertheless assumed and provided limited support for the development of a 'professional culture', embodying professional identities and values. Although this professionalism was always partial and fragile, it created the possibility of a collective identification with 'social work' and a sense of professional (rather than organisational) loyalty and commitment. The current tendencies threaten to replace this professional culture with 'corporate' identities and commitments. Current managerial discourses place a premium on creating attachments to the specific employing organisation (in the symbolic forms of its vision, mission, business plan and so on), rather than to a wider professional community. The arrival of the 'care manager' in social care has been one very visible symbol of these changes – marking the shift from social-work practitioner to a managerialised role and identity. Overlaid on other changes such as the fragmentation of the 'social-work task' and processes of de- and re-skilling, these attempts to build corporate cultures and loyalties are necessarily hostile to professional commitments since professionalism threatens to transcend corporate concerns in pointing to objectives, ethics and values beyond the organisation's core business.

These changes are condensed in what is perceived as the 'professional crisis' of social work, which is itself one aspect of the wider crisis of the bureau-professional regime that dominated the old welfare state. The changes dislocate the old terrains of conflict over

the 'role of social work' and all its attendant ambiguities. They
disrupt the points of tension, the alliances and the very languages
through which those conflicts have been fought. How can one
struggle over what a 'client-centred social work' would look like
when the client has been abolished and replaced by a 'customer'?
How can commitments to 'anti-discriminatory practice' be articulated with a managerial agenda which is dominated by the quest for
efficiency? The old points of leverage have been marginalised, even
where they have not disappeared altogether, to be replaced by
competition, corporate visions and confusion. That multi-faceted
dislocation matters both for those who practise social work and for
those who receive it. For both, the future looks bleaker 'after social
work'.

ACKNOWLEDGEMENTS

This chapter draws heavily on collaborative work with other people
– in particular, Julie Charlesworth, Allan Cochrane, Mary Langan
and Janet Newman – and would not have been possible without them.
On the other hand, they are not responsible for the somewhat
idiosyncratic uses made of that work in this context. I am grate-
ful for comments from participants at the Keele seminar, Allan
Cochrane, Gail Lewis, Janet Newman and Larry Grossberg, which
have helped it along its way.

Chapter 4

Postmodernism, feminism and the question of difference

Fiona Williams

The aim of this chapter is to explore developments in feminist theorising in relation to other developments in social theory; in particular, the shift from Enlightenment to postmodernist thinking. The chapter is concerned with the areas of convergence and divergence in feminist and postmodernist theories and the insights each offers. In particular, it interrogates the concept of difference which is central to developments in both these theoretical approaches. It asks what we understand by difference and where that understanding fits into, on the one hand, a commitment to resist forms of dominance and subordination, and on the other, current developments in welfare. The chapter also carries a sub-plot, and that is that we have to understand feminism (in all its varieties) as both part of the impulse of the Enlightenment and as part of the critique of Enlightment thinking. As such, feminism, in common with other theories of 'otherness' stemming from the so-called 'new' social movements, has the capacity to struggle through the pure relativist impasse which some postmodernist thinking has reached and, in that process, perhaps to touch some of the dogged materialist universalism of class-centric theory. What I also hope to do in this chapter is to elaborate some conceptual background to inform anti-oppressive practices in social work.

Commenting upon the two positions presented above – dogged materialism and pure relativist postmodernism – the philosopher Kate Soper has commented wryly:

> The caricature presents us on the one side with the dogged metaphysicians, a fierce and burly crew, stalwartly defending various bedrocks and foundations by means of an assortment of trusty but clankingly mechanical concepts such as 'class',

'materialism', 'humanism', 'literary merit', 'transcendence' and so forth. Obsolete as these weapons are, they have the one distinct advantage that in all the dust thrown up by the flailing around with them, their wielders do not realise how seldom they connect with the opposition. On the other side stands the opposition, the feline ironists and revellers in relativism, dancing light-heartedly upon the waters of difference, deflecting all foundationalist blows with an adroitly directed ludic laser beam. Masters of situationist strategy, they side-step the heavy military engagement by refusing to do anything but play.

(Soper, 1993: 19)

While it would seem preferable to be accused of being a playful feline ironist rather than a mechanical materialist clanker, it is nevertheless necessary, in my view, to ensure that this irony is melded with some of the ire and iron most associated with the mechanical clankers. If this chapter represents an attempt to do this, then it also represents a synthesis of the ideas of others. In the first two parts – on the shifts from Enlightenment to postmodernist thinking and the shifts within feminism – I draw on the work of Michèle Barrett (1991), Ann Philipps (1993), and Barrett and Phillips (1992), Rosemary Pringle and Sophie Watson (1992), Judith Squires (1993) and Anna Yeatman (1994). I suggest that the main developments in feminist thinking (in Britain and the United States) from the 1970s to the 1990s came from, on the one hand, internal political debates within feminism, especially, but not exclusively, around the question of differences between women and, on the other, from external (though not wholly) theoretical and political developments especially around post-structuralism and the work of Foucault, Derrida and Lacan. I want to begin by explaining, briefly and in general terms, this second development.

THE SHIFT TO A POSTMODERNIST PARADIGM

The historical and philosophical roots of modernist thinking lie in the ideals of the Enlightenment. These are characterised by a constellation of ideas: a view of the subject as powerful and self-consciously political; a belief in reason and rationality; and a belief in social and economic progress through, in particular, grand schemes of change (Barrett and Phillips, 1992: 5). It is possible to imagine this as a description of social work and the discipline of social administration at the beginning of the twentieth century. Such ideas also shaped the underpinnings of nineteenth- and twentieth-century political and social theories. While the theories of Marx, Durkheim, Weber or the functionalists, such as Parsons, may carry quite different political implications, they have in common a focus upon grand theory – the meta-narrative – upon the determining nature of the structure of society, upon progress, whether evolutionary or revolutionary, and upon society as a totality. Running through such theories is also a quest for a universal truth, and underlying such theories is a way of analysing the world through oppositional categories: ruling class/working class; man/woman; culture/nature; science or reason/emotion.

It is important to remember that feminism emerged as part of and out of the Enlightenment. One only has to think of Dorothea in George Eliot's novel *Middlemarch* to see the struggle for women to be equal to men – to be allowed into the public world of social, political and economic progress, to be seen as reasoning and powerful subjects, to play more than a bit-part in the grand scheme. At the same time, however, feminism also provided one of the profoundest critiques of Enlightenment thinking. But more of that later, for post-structuralist theory in particular (and by that I mean that body of social theory influenced by the French writers Foucault and Derrida) and postmodernism, in general, have also posed a major challenge to the social and political theories that are rooted in the Enlightenment. They have done this in five clear ways.

First, rather than understanding the subject as conscious, rational and coherent, postmodernism has emphasised much more the role of the unconscious and the fragmented nature of the self, pointing out that there are a myriad of different subjectives and different realities. Derrida calls this 'the death of Man'. (It should be said that postmodernism is not – indeed, cannot be in its own terms – a homogeneous set of ideas: I am talking here of general trends and emphases.) Second, it has challenged the emphasis upon universalism by emphasising both the relativity and the constructedness of knowledge or so-called 'truth'. There are no overarching truths, no scientific answers – for these are only partial knowledges constructed in the specifics of time and place, allegedly.

Third, it has challenged the materialist, determinist and structuralist mode of explanation for social phenomena. Postmodernism represents a shift away from finding a cause for social phenomena, a shift away from fundamentalist or essentialist thinking towards an exploration of the meanings of social phenomena and how they constitute themselves through those meanings. Here the emphasis is not on facts or evidence but upon representation, symbols and language, for it is through these that meaning is constructed. In this way, the focus is not on the cause of social problems (poverty, the so-called 'culture of dependency', or whatever) but upon how social problems come to be defined and constructed in the way they do and, at least for some post-structuralists such as Foucault, how they and the policies they engender become part of a complex of localised power relations. Meanings are articulated through discourses. The use of the term 'discourse' is a self-conscious attempt to move away from both the sharp distinction between ideology (ideas) and materiality (things) and the Marxist understanding in which ideology, after all is said and done, is determined by materiality. Instead, 'discourse' allows us to understand the complex ways in which ideologies and materiality are bound together. The emphasis has moved then, as Michele Barrett points out, from things to words (1992: 201).

Fourth, whereas the social and political theories of the twentieth century anticipated the development of societies in a stage-by-stage movement of progress, postmodernism emphasises much more the specifics of time and space, the contingencies and constellations of specific moments. And finally, the shift has been away from dualist thinking – the ordering of the social into oppositional or binary categories – towards an understanding of the multi-faceted nature of identities and phenomena. The emphasis is not so much on the difference between subjects (male/female) but upon understanding how those differences are constructed and how the categories ('man', 'woman') are themselves constituted through difference. Identities are not, in this way, seen as fixed, but ambiguous, fluid and unstable, changing with the shifting power relations of time and place.

Now, to go back to the question of feminism's part in all of this, it is possible to see that feminism seems to share with postmodernism some of the attributes I have described. It, too, provided a critique of the universalism inherent in social and political thought through its exposure of universal thinking as male-centred, whether in Marx, Freud or Friedman. It, too, challenged the oppositional categories of 'man' and 'women' (at least, in so far as they upheld the *status quo* of inequality), of public and private, arguing that these divisions were constructed not in God's or nature's image, but in the power-imagery of men. Feminism, too, was suspicious of the meta-narrative, preferring to give voice to women's narratives of their experiences of power relations in localised sites of struggle – in bedrooms and kitchens, shopfloors, doctor's surgeries, schools and streets. Feminism insisted upon the power of image and representation to shape the materiality of women's lives; it insisted upon the power of ideology to construct women as Good Mothers and Bad Mothers, as Virgins and Whores, each image complexly nuanced with the differences of class, race, ethnicity, age, disability and sexuality. It showed how these images surfaced in the texts of policies and in the practices of those who implemented them. Feminism was among those who initiated the search for conceptual tools to capture a notion of male power – patriarchy, the relative autonomy of masculinist ideology, whatever – that was denied in the theories of economic determinism. Feminism offered its own critique of modernity: it challenged the faith in reason over emotion and the implicit masculinity of the rational, coherent subject. It, too, contributed to the 'death of Man'; feminism provided women with a different route to a man's heart – this time straight through the hanky pocket with a laser-sharp mind. However, although feminism shares these developments in its thinking with postmodernism, there are also some important divergences. Before looking at those, I want to explain how feminism itself has undergone its own 'paradigm shift'.

DEVELOPMENTS IN FEMINIST THINKING

I mentioned earlier that changes within feminism over the last twenty years have been influenced by both its own internal debates and the development of post-structuralism. I want to suggest that there are three important areas of internal debate which have affected feminism. The first is around the question of differences between women. The second is a reassessment of sexual (and bodily) difference – that is, the understanding and implications of the difference between women and men, especially in terms of strategies based upon an assumption of women as equal to men, or an assumption of women as different from men. The third is the exploration of subjectivity – what it means to be a 'woman' – not simply in terms of external representations of femininity, but in terms of women's own point in the construction of their identities and the part that the unconscious (say, desire) may play in this.

Michele Barrett and Ann Phillips (1992) have outlined some of the key features in what they see as a 'paradigm shift' in the feminism of the 1970s compared with those of the 1990s (ibid.: 2–9). Briefly, they suggest that feminisms of the 1970s were characterised by a search for the cause of women's oppression: whether this was capitalism, patriarchy, capitalist patriarchy, patriarchal capitalism, or dual systems of exploitation and oppression, or whether it was patriarchy as male control over women's sexuality, fertility or labour. Second, whatever the cause, it was deemed to lie within the social structure. Third, a clear distinction was drawn between sex – representing the bare necessities of bodily difference – and gender – the socially constructed attributes of femininity and masculinity. This consensus, Barrett and Phillips argue, was broken up by three debates I mentioned above: the issue of differences between women, an attempt to re-evaluate women positively as 'different', and third, and associatedly, an attempt to understand the construction of femininity as more than an ideology foisted upon women, but as something which women themselves construct, in positive and powerful ways. These debates were also crystallised by the development of postmodernist ideas which were themselves pursuing similar lines of enquiry – into difference and the ambiguity of identity and subjectivity. I want to use Barrett and Phillips' description of the paradigm shift to focus more closely on the question of difference. The feminisms of the 1970s were concerned with a search for an explanation of the social causes of women's oppression. Within this, differences between women and differences between men and women were regarded as minimal. The emphasis tended towards the solidarity to be drawn from the commonalities of oppression that women shared – as women. (This issue is, however, the subject of competing interpretations and contrasting memories – see Griffin *et al.*, 1994.) The minimising of differences between men and women also seemed to be an important theoretical basis from which to argue for equity with men. In so far as differences were pursued, they tended to focus more on differences drawn from different political approaches – socialist, radical and liberal feminisms – rather than upon differences obtaining to women's personal identities or social positionings. And these political differences were marked by different views as to the cause (capitalism, patriarchy) and major site (work, family, sexuality, culture) of women's oppression and therefore, of course, as to the long-term strategies these implied. Nevertheless, the here-and-now strategies of the 1970s united different feminists around demands for equality – in pay, education and training, over reproductive rights and over improved public services (child-care, and so on) in order to meet women's needs.

The 1980s saw a number of different challenges to these ideas and strategies. One was a twist upon the notion of women as different from men. Many of the grass-roots campaigns of women during the 1970s and 1980s were based on developing alternative approaches to tackling women's problems or political issues – women's refuges, well-women health groups, the anti-nuclear campaign at Greenham Common. Through these women began, in contrast to earlier concerns about women as 'other' through male oppression, to present this otherness as a positive identity: women's differences from men – their commitments to care, to emotion, to nature were not to be minimised but to be celebrated. This process produced two important shifts: not only did it turn the notion of women's difference from men on its head, it also proposed that the basis for women's political identity was not so much rooted in women's shared oppression by men but in women's shared identity as different from men. It marked, in other words, a shift towards political identity rooted in difference. At the same time, however, while this development in feminism strengthened the challenge feminism had made to the universal pretensions inherent in Western political thought, it too was challenged for the universal pretensions inherent in its own notions of sisterhood. And it was this challenge that was most powerfully made by black feminists in the 1980s. The arguments within this challenge are now well documented (Carby, 1982; Phoenix, 1986; Williams, 1989; Hill-Collins, 1991). The main point is that black feminists forcibly raised the issue of the need to acknowledge the ways in which existing social divisions reconstitute women's experiences of the world, and that the category 'woman' is itself differentiated by class, race, ethnicity, disability, sexuality and age (to name but a few).

These two developments around difference were significant processes in the paradigm shift of feminism. First, the turn in the understanding of women's sexual difference has opened up the equality/difference debate (see, for example, work on women and citizenship – Philips, 1993; Lister, 1993), but has also given rise to work concerned with the significance of the body and understanding of our own embodiment – issues which are as significant for an understanding of health care as for an understanding of cultural representation. Weaving in and out of this development has been the work of Foucault, for whom the body is an important site of power and control.

The critique from black feminists around differences between women further reinforced the development of a politics of identity; that is, the idea that political identity is rooted in difference. But it also challenged the theoretical limitations in feminism's search for a cause of women's oppression. For if no single determinant could be found for women's oppression, then neither could one be found for oppression through racism. Imperialism, colonialism, the political economy of migration, forms of exclusion and religious and ethnic dominance all played a part. The very complexity of the interplay of these within patriarchal societies and capitalist economies in constituting black women's experiences seemed to make the search for a cause too obscure. What was more significant was an analysis of this complex interplay that the differences of race, class, gender, sexuality, age and disability wrought upon women's experiences.

This shift, I would argue, is an important one and, in common with the shift to postmodernist thinking, although it poses some problems, provides us with the opportunity to develop more complex enquiries into the relationship between identity, subjectivity, subject position and political agency and the way these relate to welfare discourses and how, in their turn, these discourses shape the materiality of people's lives. By breaking up analytical categories in this way – into identity, subjectivity, position and agency – it also enables us to detach ourselves from the categories and meanings imposed by policy-makers, welfare managers or (some) social researchers, and to pursue what the categories of 'single mother', 'the old', 'the disabled', and so on, mean to those who inhabit them.

So far it is clear that some of the theoretical developments with feminism both contributed to and were influenced by the shifts in social theory. However, at the same time, there have been some areas of divergence. In her book *The Politics of Truth* Michele Barrett argues that one significant area of divergence is around feminism's insistence upon humanism. In other words, feminism, in its concern with women's oppression, still keeps in the frame the notion of the subject as a political agent, however unstable, fragmented and unconnected. What is important, then, is to develop a more complex understanding of this agency in its relationship to identity, subjectivity and position. In principle, we could argue that feminism, in straddling the modern/postmodern divide, has the capacity to develop this issue of humanism (and associated issues of ethics/values, solidarity and justice) which are denied or repressed by the more relativist perspectives within postmodernism, as well as some of the more heavy-handed and social control-focused applications of Foucault's work. And it has the capacity to develop them in such a way that it takes account of notions of instability, difference and contingency highlighted by postmodernism. This is a possibility raised by Razia Aziz when she calls for a 'feminism of difference'. On the one hand, she recognises that the importance of postmodernist thinking is that it can 'save identity from "mummifying" by challenging us self-consciously to deconstruct our identities' (Aziz, 1992: 304), but she also says,

> An anti-humanist stance on always deconstructing subjectivity ignores political context and the importance of identity in resistance. The assertion that identity is a process people can relate to because it reclaims agency and makes them feel powerful. But the focus on language and subjectivity which divorces them from material forces also divorces theory from some of the things that affect people most severely.
>
> (Ibid.)

I am arguing here for a theoretical development which takes account of the conceptual markers of postmodernist thinking – particularism, difference, relativism, contingency, fragmentation, (de)constructionsism – and works out their relationship to their modernist precursors – universalism, commonality, truth, pattern, structure, essentialism, determinism. This is not to set up a new range of dualisms; rather, it is to do the opposite and understand the spaces for movement in between. As an example of this I now explore some of the political problems associated with the question of 'difference'.

THE QUESTION OF DIFFERENCE

Feminism based on black, lesbian and disabled politics has pointed to the need to deconstruct the category 'woman', in order to understand the complex and inter-connected range of identities and subject positions through which women's experiences are constituted, as well as the way these also change over time and place. Avtar Brah captures this complexity in writing about young black women in Britain. She says:

African-Caribbean and Asian women in Britain seem to be
constructing diasporic identities that simultaneously assert a sense
of belonging to the locality in which they have grown up, as well
as proclaiming a 'difference' that references the specificities of the
historical experience of being black, Asian or Muslim. And all of
these are changing subject positions. The precise ways and with
what outcome such identities are mobilised is variable. But they
speak as 'British' identities with all the complexity, contradiction
and difficulty this term implies.

(Brah, 1993: 26)

Marking out and deconstructing the complexities of difference is
important, but what are the political implications of such a focus?
What do we mean by difference? Are all differences the same? Are
all differences to be celebrated? To what end is difference claimed?
If we go on recognising differences within differences, are we left
with any meaningful category of 'woman'? Can groups whose
political identities are rooted in their difference move beyond their
own specific interests? Are notions of commonality, solidarity and
consensus relevant at all?

In order to pursue these questions I want to distinguish between
three different political understandings of the notions of difference.
This is informed by similar categorisations made by Barrett (1987)
and Brah (1992). I have called the three 'diversity', 'difference' and
'division'. By *diversity* I mean difference claimed upon a shared
collective experience which is specific and not necessarily associated
with a subordinated or unequal subject position – a shared language,
nationality regional origin, age, generation, sexual identity, marital
status, physical condition and so on.

Difference denotes a situation where a shared collective experi-
ence/identity – say, around or combining gender, ethnicity, sexuality, religion, disability – forms the basis for resistance against the
positioning of that identity as subordinate. By *division* I mean the
translation of the expression of a shared experience into a form of
domination. This is where a dominant subject position – being white,
British, heterosexual, a man – forms an identity which protects a
privileged position. At its most extreme level the British National
Party represents such a type of difference.

These are not fixed categories. The first category could become
the second or third. The women's movement in Britain in the 1970s
is a clear example of 'difference' which then became accused of

moving into 'division'. On the other hand, one group could generate the expression of all three types. In Britain, for some local Muslim communities the commitment to Islamic conventions represents a form of expression of a shared cultural and religious tradition (diversity). However, at times – as in Bradford in 1993 when there was a protest against the denial of parental choice in secondary schooling – it can become the basis for resistance against racist schooling (difference). At the same time, adherence to cultural or religious conventions can also constitute a way of maintaining old forms of male, religious power in the community (division) (Patel, 1990). This kind of movement between forms of difference needs to be seen as constant, for, within this last example, the very meaning of culture is transformed with each reconstruction.

These distinctions may go some way to understanding the differences within difference, and we might even go so far as to say that we would be 'for' some and 'against' others. But there remains a more complex question – does the expression of difference inevitably lead to a form of closure or exclusivity which in itself prevents such groups from moving beyond their specific interests and therefore from recognising any commonalities they may share with others?

In other words, does the process of asserting a common identity as one which is forged in its specific difference mean that, first, other facets of a group's/person's identity are obscured, and that such identities become frozen into an essentialist category of difference? After all, these were the experiences of the women's movement. Its focus upon a specific category – 'woman' – obscured other identities and positions women had and, second, some women's claim to difference – closeness to nature, emotion – overlapped uncomfortably with right-wing notions of women as biologically essentialist wives and mothers.

Yet, in order to claim difference we need to fix it, freeze it and understand it through and through. So perhaps the issue is whether, in fixing upon a difference, a group does so with a consequence of freezing the power relations around it, or challenging and changing those power relations, or securing the power within those relations and structures. I am suggesting that it is on the basis of the second that difference can be used creatively to move beyond particular interests: in fact, it is this very process of challenge that becomes the commonality that groups may share. It provides an environment in which temporarily frozen identities may melt and run into one another.

However, this is not a straightforward process: the temporary fixing and claiming of difference may often involve steps back as well as, or before, steps forward. In spite of this linear metaphor, I want to imply that the notion of contingency is an important one in this context. Talking about the category of 'woman' Joan Scott observes:

> Political strategies will then rest on analyses of the utility of certain arguments in certain discursive contexts without, however, invoking absolute qualities for women or men. There are moments when it makes sense for mothers to demand consideration for their social role, and contexts within which motherhood is irrelevant to women's behaviour; but to maintain that motherhood is womanhood is to obscure the differences that make that choice possible.
>
> (Scott, 1992: 262–3)

So our political identities are not fixed or rigid or set in stone. Yet, for the purpose of consolidation they may have to be held as fixed, temporarily frozen. What is important is where they are then taken – down paths of resistance or dominance. The fragmentation of politics involves a constant freezing and melting and reconstituting of identity. At the same time, we cannot assume that commonalities (as women, or among different groups) exist, nor can we override differences with a false consensus. But it is through the process of knowing, acknowledging and understanding the complex relations of power in which we are all caught and the differences they create that we can, from time to time, reach the commonalities we share. As Michele Barrett and Anne Phillips say, these commonalities represent a goal and not a given (Barrett and Phillips, 1992: 9).

THE DISCURSIVE CONTEXT OF DIFFERENCE IN WELFARE

Such struggles over difference outlined in the previous section do not occur in a vacuum but in a context in which there are competing meanings and discourses around notions of diversity and difference. 'Cultural diversity' might be one such discourse, with its understanding of the potential for the peaceful coexistence of different cultural groups. However, this notion often ignores the external relations of dominant and subordinate cultural groups (indeed, often the word 'ethnic' only ever applies, in Britain to those whose cultures lie outside or subordinate to the dominant white Christian culture). It also implies a static and essentialist notion of cultures which 'coexist' rather than inter-relate and transform one another. Similarly, while it may be helpful in legitimating other cultures, it may obscure the relations of power within those cultures and fix people too readily to an identity they may hold with great ambivalence. This is one example of such a discourse, but I want to look more closely at the discourses of diversity which operate within recent developments in welfare.

There are three key ways in which the notion of diversity or difference is mobilised within social welfare in Britain in the 1990s. The first is an individualist notion of diversity which operates through choice. The second is managerialist and focuses upon the management of differentiated needs. The third is anti-discriminatory and mobilises difference as political identity. The individualist approach to diversity has emerged from the New Right's development of the mixed economy of welfare in Britain. Notions of diversity and difference are mobilised to counter the monopolistic and universalistic characteristics of the Keynesian welfare state. They enter welfare discourses in two main ways – through the pluralism of welfare providers and through the diversity of choice offered to welfare users through the mechanism of the market. The opening up of the voluntary and private sectors is supposed to create a diversity of provision which is able to meet the diverse choices and needs of the population. In this approach the notions of diversity and difference are quite unexplained: different needs and different choices are collapsed into one and are supposed to find their expression through the market. The welfare consumer in this scenario is totally individualised – few distinctions are made between carers and people who receive care, between pupils and parents, or between the economic constraints on parts of the population. In so far as differences of a less individualised nature are acknowledged, these are often ascribed to essential behavioural or cultural difference. For example, in some places the provision of Muslim schools has been supported on the grounds of recognising essential cultural differences in the population. Differences in types and quality of school have also been defended on the basis of differences in the 'cultural aspirations' of parents. Differences, too, between those users who are compelled to use welfare services (claimants, clients) and those who are not are explained in terms of the 'dependency culture' of the first group. In this approach, then, the market is seen to encourage diverse provision and the expression of differentiated needs. Differences within the population are seen as natural or voluntaristic. Unequal needs are interpreted as the expression of the constructed provision of morally inferior choices (the choice to be dependent upon the state), which in turn create groups identified as social problems – single parents, scroungers, 'yobs', and so on.

The managerialist notion of diversity and difference has entered welfare discourses largely through the 1990 NHS and Community Care Act and the restructuring of health and social care. Much of the implementation of recent policy centres upon the introduction of a 'needs-based' service, where the separation of the roles of purchasers and providers has been accompanied by a requirement that purchasers assess the needs of potential service-users on a needs-led basis. Although this breaks with past practice where services were based on providers' definitions of need, here needs, and the diversity and differences of those needs, are again largely recognised on individual terms: individuals have different needs for which individual care packages can be organised. Again, while this breaks with past practices which emphasised uniformity of need rather than individuality of circumstance – financial, physical, support and so on – the approach to the definition of difference still lies firmly rooted in professional or managerially defined categories – old, sick, at risk, disabled, people who are dangerous to themselves or others, vulnerable and so on. Even the category 'ethnic minorities', having eventually achieved recognition, has found itself wedged uncomfortably into a rather discrete, essentialist and managed client group. Nevertheless, there may exist within this approach spaces for the collective articulation of differentiated needs in which different patterns and meanings of diversity and difference emerge; for example, through local needs audits (see Percy-Smith and Sanderson, 1992), or through the collective organisation of service-users. This will depend largely on the strength of the third discourse of diversity, discussed below, but in general within the context of efficiency and economy individuals are increasingly being displaced into administrative categories – the elderly, children with special needs and so on – and the assessment of needs may become yet another assessment of means or of physical or mental incapacities.

The third discourse of diversity and difference has emerged from the demands for equal opportunities policies and for anti-

discriminatory practices, especially around gender, race and disability and, in some places, sexuality. These have been important in
raising issues of discrimination within welfare organisations and,
where they have been translated into anti-discriminatory practice, for
service-users. Along with the development of equal opportunities
has been the emergence since the 1980s of local, national and
international movements of the collective organisation of welfare
constituents based outside the statutory services. For example, the
disability movement comprises a range of disabled people's groups
such as the Union of the Physically Impaired Against Segregation
(UPIAS) or the British Council of Disabled People (BCODP);
'Survivors Speak Out' exists for users of psychiatric services and
'People First' for the development of self-advocacy for people with
learning difficulties. These groups have their own individual histories but they also have their political roots in the emancipatory
movements around gender and 'race' oppressions. Their practice has
also been influenced by some of the self-help welfare initiatives to
emerge from these movements. In terms of the categories of
difference discussed in the previous section, what is interesting about
these groups is the fact that they have grasped the administrative
categories (or subject positions) imposed upon them by policy-
makers, administrators and practitioners and translated these into
political identities and new subjectivities. However, for some groups
this process has moved in the opposite direction. As mentioned
above, claims for difference and struggles by black and minority
ethnic groups against racist practices have sometimes been appropriated within the new social services management as part of a
strategy of managing difference, using the expertise of black social
workers.

CONCLUSION

I propose that one of the key areas of contestation within health and
social care is over these meanings – and the practices associated with
them – of diversity and difference. I have suggested that at least three
discourses of diversity and difference have emerged in the restructuring of welfare: one based upon the exercise of consumer
choice within the diversity of the marketised mixed economy; a
second based upon the management of diverse needs, articulated
individually by consumers but assessed and re-routed through
administrative categories and financial stringencies. The third is

rooted in political identity and acts as a challenge to existing power relations and a re-appropriation of imposed administrative categorisations. In practice, whereas the emphasis in recent policy upon services sensitive to needs creates, rhetorically at least, the space for the articulation of needs, its practices and procedures of assessment and its context of tightening budgets mean that the political claiming of difference can be shifted back into an individualised problem group or a managed category. The capacity to resist this shift depends upon the ends to which difference is claimed – the issue discussed in the third part of this chapter. Some of the difficulties associated with the development of equal opportunities can be analysed better within both the understanding of the different meanings of claims for difference and an understanding of competing welfare discourses of diversity. The shift in emphasis from equality of opportunities to 'control of quality' is part of the context in which equal opportunities policies and units have been displaced or dispensed with. However, some attention should also be paid to the tendency of equal opportunities policies to organise around discrete categories of oppression – to 'freeze' differences – which, within the context of financial constraints, has slipped all too easily into competing claims of need. It has also inhibited the recognition of the inter-relatedness of oppression and to a tendency to ossify difference as rigid and essential and thereby to a difficulty in linking common needs (for improved general services) to particular interests (for the meeting of specific needs). The capacity of the new welfare mobilisations around gender, race, sexuality and disability to generate a resistance and/or an alternative to the current rhetorically named 'needs-led' approach will partly depend upon their capacity to 'freeze' into solidarities of specificity and 'melt' into loosely attached units of commonality, according to the political contingencies of time and space. This chapter has argued that postmodernist thinking has offered us important insights into the understanding of these specificities of time and space and the fragmented nature of the self. However, in so far as feminist thinking has also struggled through these new complexities and conceptualisations it has, by and large, still retained its commitment to challenge the unequal power relations inherent within them. And that, too, is important.

Chapter 5

Surface and depth in social-work practice

David Howe

Social work's theories and practices reflect the times in which they live. In a deep sense, social work is defined by the evolving relationship between the state and the individual. Any changes in definition of either the political or the personal therefore result in shifts in how we understand that domain in which the state and the individual meet. This domain or discourse we now know as the *social*. Recent upheavals in the philosophy and politics surrounding welfare have resulted in redefinitions of both the *social* and those who work-the-*social*, rightly called social workers. In the wake of such changes, social work's knowledge base and practice repertoire have also experienced major alterations in their character.

I want to argue that in these new political and cultural contexts many of social work's theories and practices have become analytically more shallow and increasingly performance-orientated. The concept of modernity will prove useful in helping us to understand the rise of the social worker in the nineteenth century. It will allow us to track her evolution from diagnostic caseworker to care manager, from applied social scientist to service coordinator.

Modernity has faced two crises, each brought about by perceived excesses in one or other of its two defining dimensions of liberty and discipline (Wagner, 1994). The first crisis witnessed growing misery and social unrest suffered under the worst features of nineteenth-century liberalism with its heavy emphasis on human *freedom* and individual autonomy. The solution to these problems of social disorder led to attempts to *discipline* and regulate social life. Social work, along with other forms of collective action in the emerging welfare state, formed as part of this disciplining process. But by the 1960s, there were growing feelings amongst New Right radical liberals that collectivism had gone too far. The welfare state was thought to be stifling the individual and individualism.

The fate of social work in this second crisis of modernity is particularly intriguing when it is remembered that social work's traditional characteristics formed in the wake of modernity's first crisis. How, we might ask, is social work faring in this new political climate which arose in reaction to the very social philosophy which helped define social work and saw it as a central part of welfare collectivism? What form does social work take when it no longer finds itself in a 'discourse' of discipline but rather one of radical liberalism? We shall explore these questions by examining the concept of modernity and the tensions that it generates.

MODERNITY

The seventeenth century and the Enlightenment witnessed profound changes in the way the physical and the social worlds were understood and approached. No longer were nature and society taken as divinely ordained; no longer was the truth of things to be revealed by studying the word of God. Nature could be investigated and fathomed by the power of human reason and rational enquiry. Human beings could examine and determine the principles upon which the physical world was based. It was recognised that there were laws of nature and that they were, in principle, knowable. Nature was underpinned by deep, universal regularities. The behaviour and appearance of the physical world could therefore be explained by determining the order that lies at the heart of nature. And once the principles and mechanisms were understood, nature itself could then be controlled, disciplined, exploited and fashioned to suit the needs and interests of men and women. The world was no longer God-given; it was to be 'man-made'. Human *reason* would lead to the truth of things, and not divine *revelation*.

Within the modern vision, rational men and women need no longer occupy and accept a fixed place in the divine order. They could *liberate* themselves from nature and the social order and so control their own destiny. No external authority, divine or secular, had the right or the power to limit that freedom. Modern times begin with the articulation of a *discourse of liberation* in which freedom and autonomy became recognised as a basic, unalienable human right (Wagner, 1994: 5). Modernity therefore becomes characterised by a strange and strained mix of freedom and control; liberty and discipline; knowledge and responsibility. Human beings are capable of shaping the world to suit their own interests, but by the same token they remain responsible for whatever kind of world they create. Once people recognised that they could *act* upon the world and that they were no longer passive players in the 'great chain of being', human beings experienced the modern condition of freedom and choice on the one hand and responsibility and insecurity on the other.

The scientific and political revolutions ushered in by the Enlightenment had a profound affect on the individual's sense of self and social identity. Although human beings had become released from the divine order and gained moral independence under the liberating powers of modernity, these times also meant that there was an ever-present threat of anarchy and chaos. With mass movements out of rural communities and into anonymous cities, the social contexts within which people's *identities* had traditionally formed and into which their sense of self had been firmly embedded suffered major disruptions. Uncertainty about one's fate and place in society increased under such dislocations. The social unrest and behavioural disorder which this induced became of growing concern throughout the nineteenth century. It seemed that the unbridled freedom of some was producing a lack of freedom and scale of misery for others that would be the undoing of the very social order which was supposed to support the autonomous individual.

In social and political terms, the late nineteenth century represented modernity's first crisis. In its pursuit of freedom and truth, the modern project seemed to have precipitated great swathes of misery and disorder across large tracts of social life. There was no doubt that the impact of an unregulated liberal economic market was producing poverty, degradation and despair on a massive scale.

The growth of the social sciences and the steady emergence of the welfare state between the 1890s and the 1960s were a direct response to the recognition that if widespread personal well-being was to be achieved, social planning and state intervention based on systematically acquired social knowledge would have to be developed. Social provisions would enable people to be protected 'from the cradle to the grave'. Solidity and certainty needed to be re-established into the social fabric (Wagner, 1994: 59). Under organised modernity, individuals would become re-embedded in the new, stable social order.

The integration of the masses and the working classes required new forms of social organisation based on *collective action*.

Throughout this period of 'organised modernity', the unfettered principle of liberty was to be steadily curbed and contained by a growing sense of collective responsibility, state control and social management. The state began to appear as that political form which sought to contain, discipline and regulate modernity's constant demand to respect the individual's right to absolute freedom. There was growing acceptance by 'communitarians' that the fate of many individuals was not the result of personal action but is the product of larger, impersonal forces against which the individual remains helpless. Only collective action could deal with social problems. And with the growth and spread of these socially organised practices, the individual became re-integrated into a world experienced as less uncertain, more predictable and more secure.

The social sciences therefore arose to do with society what the physical sciences had done with nature: explain it, order it, control it and improve it. The concept and practice of 'social engineering' became a possibility. In emulating the success of the physical sciences, the social and political sciences sought to develop methods of rational enquiry which would reveal fundamental truths about personal and social life upon which notions of the good society and the creation of order might be based. As theories and practices of the 'collective' grew and as collective actions became more widespread, the social sciences gained in both self-understanding and the ability to interpret social life. The difficult and the distressed, including their relationship to social structures, could be explained. So, as well as progress in the physical sciences, it was possible to conceive of progress in human affairs: the social world, too, could be made better. In its grand form, the project of modernity was seen as a programme 'to liberate human beings from their subjection to nature, from unchosen ties to others, and from contradictions within themselves. After all, modernity is a rebellion against fate and ascription' (Wagner, 1994: 45). The social sciences arose to theorise and service modernity (Bauman, 1992: 54) and to bring about rational control over social development and a sense of moral progress in political life.

THE FORMATION OF SOCIAL WORK

The disruptions experienced as the old social orders broke down under the conflict between the coercing powers of industrialisation on the one hand and the rhetoric of political rights and freedoms on the other meant that somehow attention had to be paid to the relationship between the condition of the individual and the maintenance of the social order. Social work therefore formed in the tension between the political and the personal and began to take on most of its general characteristics during the second half of the nineteenth century. It was one of a number of occupations which arose as the state and various collective associations (charities, trade unions, voluntary organisations) showed increasing concern and interest in the experiences and behaviour of individuals who either suffered distress or caused distress (Donzelot, 1979).

The 'social' was defined as that area in which personal relationships (family life, child-rearing practices, interpersonal behaviour) became of interest to the state, and the state's attitude to personal behaviour became relevant to the individual. The 'social' emerged as an area between the private and the public, a field in which the state penetrated the world of private relationships. It was a discourse in which it became possible to define and represent the strong and the rich to the weak and the poor and vice versa (Philp, 1979). In one and the same act *social* workers became a group who could both judge the actions of others *and* seek to treat those actions. Social work formed under the double perspective of control *and* cure, as it embraced both the judicial and the therapeutic in single acts of intervention (Donzelot, 1979; Parton, 1994a; Howe, 1994). And to help them carry out these interventions, social workers turned to the social and psychological sciences, applying their insights and explanations to social problems and problem people. Social work, therefore, formed and was thoroughly immersed in one of modernity's key projects – to bring discipline and order, progress and improvement to the human condition.

In its traditional range of theories and practices, social work has assumed that there is a deeper order of reality which lies beneath individual behaviour and social life. It is the working of these social and psychological regularities which govern what people say and do, experience and understand. Surface appearances are said to be the external manifestation of these underlying principles. If these internal mechanisms and the laws which govern them can be discovered, it then becomes possible to (1) understand and explain people and their behaviour, (2) control and improve people and their behaviour, and (3) treat and fix those examples of behaviour which appear to be either not working or not functioning appropriately. To such ends, social workers have studied and sought to apply a range of psychological and sociological theories to problematic individuals, families and social situations.

SOCIAL WORK UNDER ATTACK

However, by the late 1960s and 1970s, increasing doubts were being expressed about the effectiveness of welfare provisions in controlling social unruliness and bringing about improvements in the quality of personal experience. This was modernity's second crisis (Wagner, 1994). Rises in crime, marital breakdown, drug abuse and the numbers of single parent families were all cited as examples of the welfare state's inability to deliver order, certainty and security in personal life.

Social work was in the front of the firing-line of much of the criticisms levelled at the welfare state. It was also under attack from within its own ranks. The more behaviourally inclined and scientifically minded researchers began to question social work's effectiveness. The claim was that social workers, particularly those who practised within a psychoanalytic tradition, were ineffective in treating such things as delinquency and poor parenting (for example, see Fischer, 1976). But social workers were also being arraigned by another set of theorists who saw social workers pathologising the individual rather than blaming the political system that promoted so much inequality and hardship. Social workers would be much more effective, so the claim went, if they attempted to change the social system to suit individuals rather than change individuals to fit the social system (for example, see Corrigan and Leonard 1978).

In spite of their contrasting analyses, both critiques remained firmly within the modern project. Although social work was charged with using the wrong theories and its methods appeared ineffective, there was still the belief by both protagonists that individual and social experience could be changed and improved by recognising the true, underlying cause of people's problems and difficulties. It just happened that social workers had latched on to a poor set of explanations and associated practices. In the case of the critical researchers, the recommendation was for more behaviourally orientated and task-centred practices, while for the sociologically inspired critics the argument was that social workers should take a more political and structural approach to understanding and dealing with clients and their problems.

But social workers were under attack from other directions too, and it was these assaults which proved to be the more significant, having a profound impact on the nature of social work as it evolved through the 1980s (Parton, 1994a: 24). It was not just that traditional social-work practices appeared to be ineffective; they were also accused of being intrusive and undermining of the moral fabric. For example, in some cases of sexual abuse, it was alleged that social workers had been too zealous. They had intervened and removed children from homes in which courts eventually decided that no abuse or proven abuse had occurred. Politicians and the media had no difficulty in accusing social workers of failing to remove and save children from families which were clearly violent and dangerous while at the same time criticising them for removing other children because of the profession's unhealthy obsession with and ex-aggeration of sexual abuse.

The claim was that social workers had too much power to intervene in family life without being either useful or effective. The state, it was argued, should be more reluctant to invade the privacy of family life; it should stop undermining parental responsibility. Not only should there be greater parental involvement in decisions and actions concerning children, it should be explicitly recognised that it is parents and not the state who are *responsible* for their children. Such policies manage to blend conservatism with liberalism, tradi-tional values of the patriarchal, self-reliant family with *laissez-faire* economics.

> The British Conservative Party Conference in 1990 yet again focused on the family and family issues and restated the position that while families need to stand on their own feet and take responsibility for their members, it is up to the state to make sure that they do.
>
> (Abbott and Wallace, 1992: 2)

So it seemed that social workers could be both intrusive as well as ineffective, sapping of family strengths as well as liable to make matters worse rather than better.

In other parts of the social services, too, there were parallel moves towards increasing client choice. Much of this choice was to be achieved by introducing the principles of the market place into the purchase, provision and delivery of welfare services. Throughout the health, educational and personal social services there was growing emphasis on consumer responsibility, choice, independence, indi-viduality and freedom. Social workers began to assess people for services rather than analyse their psychological and social condition. The ubiquitous and endlessly promiscuous concept of 'partnership', emphasising and encouraging the independence and legal rights of the client, appeared and found favour with both the political right and the political left, though for contrasting reasons. Where the left saw empowerment of the poor and disadvantaged, the right saw growth in personal responsibility, independence and individual choice.

LIBERTY AND DISCIPLINE

We appear, then, to be faced with an irony. Out of freedom arises the need for discipline. By the late nineteenth century, the unbridled autonomy of the individual was producing social unrest and political tension. This triggered a demand for collective action to help maintain the social order and increase the basic range of human freedoms and social goods to be enjoyed by the greatest number. The ambivalence that runs as a thread through modernity's struggles to handle both liberty and discipline is captured in the perennial attempts by sociology and political theory to deal with individual liberalism on the one hand and collective well-being on the other (Avineri and de-Shalit, 1992; Mulhall and Swift, 1992).

Towards the end of the nineteenth century and throughout most of the twentieth century until the 1980s, constraints on individual freedom had been expressed through the activities of the welfare state. There is little doubt that collective action ensured and improved the broad well-being of the majority of individuals. But it also required an intrusion into private life and a restriction on individual freedom, autonomy and personal choice to ensure the collective good and the broad emancipation of the many and not just the few. The form in which this result was achieved:

> was *collectivization*. Both from below and from above, the building of the welfare state was a major collectivizing process. It assigned the members of society to places in well-defined collectives according to age, occupational status, marital status, health status. The status definition was accompanied by expectations about behaviour opportunities and actual behaviour, and an increasing number of welfare bureaucrats and social workers of all kinds were ready to intervene should the reality deviate from expectations. The effect of the welfare state can

without doubt be seen as a standardization of social behaviour and of biographical positions. . . . By means of statistical calculation, case assessment and redistributive measures, dangers were transformed into calculable risks. . . . Calculation and assessment provided the forms for a rationalization of life that brought standardization about.

(Wagner, 1994: 98)

The apparent failures of the welfare state to guarantee safety, personal growth and improved behaviour coupled with its alleged undermining of initiative, independence and creativity has seen a swing back in the 1980s to a radical re-emphasis on modernity's other defining characteristic – human freedom. Such an emphasis is the hallmark of the 'neo-liberal', the champion of the market place, personal responsibility and choice, prepared only to recognise the individual and his or her individuality. In its extreme form, radical liberalism sees no need for external constraints or welfare experts who attempt to set boundaries around individuals and their right to be self-determining. The principal task of society is to ensure that individuals can lead autonomous lives. For the neo-liberal, it is the rational actions of individuals which guarantee that society functions most effectively and most efficiently. So, whereas modernity in the nineteenth century was only able to support the freedom and individuality of a few at the expense of the many, modernity in the late twentieth century, in declaring the failure of welfare collectivism, is able to offer freedom and the possibility of individual expression to the majority. This has allowed the development of great *plurality* in life-styles, cultural values, expressions of difference, and the steady erosion of a shared moral, aesthetic and value base. With doubts about the ability of human reason to generate universal truths and establish order and progress in human affairs, truths and values are now taken to be relative to time and place, culture and people.

It is this *fin-de-siècle* return to a philosophy which celebrates liberal values of freedom and the autonomy of the heroic individual that has coincided with the emergence of what many people call a 'postmodern' age. It appears as a response to the doubts beginning to be felt about modernity's belief that the social world is essentially both knowable and manageable and that order can be shaped by human design based on fundamental moral and scientific truths or 'meta-narratives'. The apparent failure of human reason to establish foundational truths in ethics, aesthetics and the social sciences, evidenced by a lack of success to detect any demonstrable progress in humanity's moral, social or aesthetic condition, cast doubt in the minds of many that there were transcendent, universal truths upon which human society could unambiguously be based – see Parton (1994a) and Howe (1994) for discussions of modernity and post-modernity in a social-work context. Indeed, those who have felt that they have discovered the fundamental truths – moral, political and social – by which all human beings might live have all too often seen their ideas lead, ironically, to a loss of freedom. In extreme versions of collective emancipation and social management, totalitarian regimes have arisen in which preferred truths have been imposed on the populace. Those who hold dissenting or alternative truths, must, by definition, be holding false truths. They threaten the foundation of the ideal society and so they are outlawed or eliminated. National Socialism in Nazi Germany and Eastern bloc communism can be cited as modern-day examples of rational thought, producing polit-ical truths and social engineering, leading eventually to barbaric practices. As Wright Mills (1970: 186) observed, increased reason may not make for increased freedom.

For the postmodernist, then, there are no fundamental truths. The truth is neither revealed by studying the word of God nor discovered by the power of human reason, for there is no one truth. Truth is relative to time and place. It is not *centred* in or derived from the texts of either divine authorities or human thought. Rather, the truth is *de-centred*. It arises in local *contexts*. No rational system of thought can legislate what is the truth. The truth can only be interpreted (Bauman, 1987). In his discussion of Baudrillard, Smart notes his challenge to those social analyses which employ con-ceptions of 'deep' and 'hidden' structures:

> Baudrillard suggests that there is no way around, through, or beyond the manifest, the surface. In other words there is no depth to discover, and that self-referentiality is a feature not only of language, but also increasingly of the culture of (post)modern everyday life.
>
> (1993: 123)

Our reality arises out of a restless, boundless sea of language, meaning and interpretation. And as our sense of self arises within relationships which are conducted in the medium of language, and as language carries meaning which undergoes endless interpretation, there can be no fixed or essential quality to human consciousness, the human self and to human being. We have no choice but to search for meaning, although there are no ultimate meanings to find. Therefore, notions of moral and social progress are illusory, danger-ous and restrictive. Life is necessarily contingent and uncertain.

No particular cultural group, according to the postmodernists, therefore holds the key to absolute standards of truth, beauty and moral conduct. No group has a privileged access to a universal set of transcendent values which apply to all persons in all cultures. Such truths and values can only be seen as oppressive narratives, intent on fixing everyone, everywhere in their place, usually to the benefit of the group promoting the 'true' reality. The overthrow of such meta-narratives serves to liberate the individual. Difference – in values, narratives, truths, meanings, interpretations – should be celebrated as well as tolerated. For example, the time of white, middle-class men being the sole arbiters of truth which they impose on all others has been overtaken by the recognition that other cultural groups – women, black people, disabled people – have an equal right to assert their values and views about how best to understand the world and respond to life. In the postmodern world, political pluralism replaces the single vision.

But postmodernism, described in this sense, is simply a reaction against collective attempts to impose welfare solutions based on alleged sociological, psychological and moral insights and truths. The discipline of modernity, the search for truth using human reason, and the pursuit of progress and improvement based on those truths all too often seemed to have led to constraint and uniformity. The only way to escape the standardisation of human experience is to recover that sense of freedom and free-for-all which first saw human reason assert itself against the divine will. In this outlook, my views are as valid as yours. There are no universal standards by which to judge the truth of a belief or the rightness of an action. There is faith in the creative power and energy of human beings unfettered by social contracts and communal expectations.

The reaction against the alleged failures of the practices of communitarian politics and a resurgence of the significance and vitality of the free and independent individual has had a huge impact on all aspects of political and social life. Social work and its practices have been caught up in these neo-liberal reactions against social action, communitarian values and state-led interventions based on the insights of the social sciences. As a result, social work has undergone a number of major changes in its interests and character (also see Parton, 1994a). I shall consider a number of these changes under the following three headings:

1 The performance of clients.
2 Competencies and the performance of social workers.
3 Social work in the market place.

The performance of clients

Within a radical liberal perspective, actions are judged more by their results and consequences. It is the client's performance which matters and not what causes it. 'Performativity' becomes the dominant criterion for knowledge evaluation (Wagner, 1994: 26). Behaviour is no longer analysed in an attempt to explain it. Rather, it is assessed in terms of administrative procedures, political expectations and legal obligations. Social workers now ask *what* clients do rather than *why* do they do it – a switch from causation to counting, from explanation to audit. Depth explanations based on psychological and sociological theories are superseded by surface considerations. It is the visible surface of social behaviour which concerns practitioners and not the internal workings of psychological and sociological entities. As Cohen (1985: 144) recognised, social workers become more inclined to respond to the *act* rather than treat the *actor*. Thus, a concern with *behaviour* replaces an interest in *action*.

In broad terms, we see social workers managing acts. The Probation Service, for example, has been encouraged to concentrate its efforts on helping clients assume responsibility for recognising the consequences of their criminal actions. It has been discouraged from paying too much attention to the psychological and social condition of the offender. It is thus the *offence* and not the *offender* which becomes the focus of concern as penal policy and practice have moved away from the concept of welfare towards the concept of justice.

In the swing towards libertarian-based values, clients are expected to comply and conform; they are not diagnosed, treated or cured. If they know the rules, it is up to them to decide whether or not to abide by them. They are seen as free agents, no longer determined by psychological and sociological forces. Personal responsibility, freedom and choice replace concepts of cause and determination. For

example, the roots of emotional impulsiveness in a troubled childhood do not inform the treatment meted out to people who are easily
roused to anger and violence. Rather, they are taught to 'manage'
their anger. They are not asked to reflect on *why* they feel a loss of
control or ponder its causes. The demand is that they work out *what*
to do when they begin to experience feelings of rage and aggression.
In this way they are encouraged to manage their social performance
in a fashion felt to be more acceptable.

Neo-liberal philosophies encourage social workers to see clients
as rational agents who, being fully informed of the situation, are free
to choose whether they behave or misbehave, knowing the consequences of their actions. Their political rights and autonomy are
respected, but, by the same token, there can be no excuses made or
'understandings' extended to those who 'wilfully' choose to trans-
gress. The strong assumption is that clients are capable of rational
action which they are said to take in their own best interests.

The growing role of a justice-orientated rather than welfare-
orientated law in work with children and their families has played a
large part in re-defining the character of social work. Social work's
ingenuous support of a rights-based liberalism in family work,
emphasising political rights and not psychological explanation, is
much more likely to manage distressed clients and difficult relationships by an insistence that participants keep to agreed roles. 'In
effect', observes Parton (1994a: 26) 'social workers are constituted
as managers of family life for certain sections of the population.'
Relationships are handled by legal fiat rather than by the use of
interpersonal skills and psychological understanding. The state,
reflects Mestrovic (1993: 55) can 'never be trusted to make persons
moral, only to punish lawbreakers'.

Social-work practices under the influence of neo-liberal philosophies also become ahistorical. Clients arrive, in effect, without a
history; their past is no longer of interest. It is their present and future
performance which matters. Present behaviour, which under a
welfare perspective was understood with reference to past experiences, is now assessed in terms of future expectations. The lack
of depth in the social-work assessment is therefore both spatial and
temporal. The evolution and development of individual personalities
and social structures is downplayed. Similarly, the analysis of
people's material, political and psychological states is less likely to
appear in court reports, assessments for conferences and case
records.

Causal accounts of behaviour have a narrative-like quality. Within a modernist perspective, sequences of events are held together and *explained* by the logic which underpins their appearance. To make sense of what is happening, reference has to be made to particular theoretical frameworks which seem best able to explain how one event is linked with another across space and through time. Modern novels, films and music have beginnings, middles and ends. Logical threads and connecting themes carry the story along as it develops and unfolds according to the principles which govern its moment-by-moment expression. To be able to follow the story and respond appropriately, you need to understand the patterns and relationships that determine who does what, why and when. For the modernist, beneath the buzz and the complexity there are rhythms and regularities which, once identified, hold the key to understanding and explanation.

For postmodernists, doubts about the existence of any transcendent systems of truth lead to the breakdown of causal narratives as a way of explaining things. The world is a contingent place. There are no deep patterns underpinning reality. In this sense, there is no arrow of history and progress has no direction. No one authority is able to speak *the* truth, for there is no single truth of which to speak. In the novel and the film, the absence of a clear story-line, the break-up and breakdown of conventional time sequences, and the use of several 'authors' seeing the world from multiple perspectives and offering their truths and versions of events, all recognise the arbitrary and contingent nature of any given 'reality'. In much mainstream postmodern cinema, for example, we see a concentration on the image, the event and the spectacle. In the case of some Spielberg, Rambo and Schwarzenegger films, there is no strong story-line; foreground spectacle prevails over underlying narrative (Lash, 1990: 191).

There are curious parallels here to be found in *fin-de-siècle* social work. There is a lack of organisational interest in constructing client narratives. We have already mentioned the demise of historically based analyses in some quarters. In task-focused and contract-orientated practices, immediate realities are negotiated, and definitions of what is and what is to be are agreed. Clients are not located and understood within the context of an ordered narrative; their story is not framed within a theoretical perspective whose principles govern what is said and done. Each episode of social-work intervention is discrete and unrelated to previous episodes. Work is short-term, time-limited and 'brief'. When the 'event' is over, the case is closed. If clients re-appear, a new scene opens but one which has no necessary relationship with earlier appearances. The action starts afresh each time. There is no accumulated wisdom because there are no psychological or sociological theoretical frameworks in which to order and store it. Each new encounter simply triggers a fresh set of transactions, negotiations and agreements. It is a here-and-now world; a world without history, pattern or direction. Cases do not progress; they are not required to go anywhere in the long run. In a sense it does not matter. It is literally a fiction to explain the present with reference to the past; there is no necessary connection. In the absence of authoritative texts to explain events, sense arises in the immediate 'context' where the client's behaviour, needs and responses meet the social worker's rules, resources and procedures. And out of such meetings arise agreements, tasks and time limits.

Competencies and the performance of social workers

Changes in the political outlook on welfare collectivism have directly affected social workers, what they do and how they are trained. The loss of faith in the effectiveness of welfare-orientated practices means that there is less interest in developing knowledge and skills designed to diagnose problems, carry out treatment plans, cure individuals and change social systems. Knowledge is used to help social workers collect appropriate information on clients as well as identify and classify them as particular types of service-user or problem-presenters. Having identified and classified the client, he or she is then eligible to receive a certain, prescribed response. This response may be a particular service, a required legal procedure or a certain kind of resource.

Less and less is the social worker expected, or indeed allowed, to make an independent, on-the-spot judgement or diagnosis of what is the matter. Less and less is the social worker likely to respond with a tailor-made, professional intervention based on his or her own knowledge and skills. There is no requirement to explore the causes of behaviours and situations, only the demand that they be described, identified and classified. It is the category into which the client's behaviour or condition fits which increasingly determines the response prescribed. The social worker is not encouraged to have independent thoughts but *is* required to act competently. The emphasis is on what people do rather than what people think.

The move towards identifying 'competencies' rather than professional skills is to be found in the training programmes of many occupations. There is a move from reason to rote. For example, in the case of some electronics technicians, the training for many simply involves the identification and classification of faults in electrical systems according to set routines, check-lists and formulae. Having identified and classified the faulty part, it is simply removed and replaced. There is no requirement to understand the underlying principles of electrical circuitry, never mind the theory of electromagnetism and its huge range of applications. What this means is that, although the 'competent' technician can fix routine faults by carrying out a sequence of prescribed responses, he or she is at a loss what to do if something 'out-of-the-ordinary' occurs.

Similarly, such a technician is unable to adapt, create or develop new electrical systems or devices. Without a knowledge of the underlying theory and principles, the practitioner is confined to performing surface responses according to pre-coded procedures. Information check-lists, problem categories and recommended responses do not need the knowledge, skills and discretionary powers of the autonomous professional. Good-quality practice is achieved when practitioners recognise the need for a particular 'competence' and can carry out that competence in an appropriate and efficient manner. Such practices are designed to bring about reliable responses of a consistent quality in a predictable, fixed task environment. In social work, this presupposes that the work is amenable to categorisation and susceptible to routine responses. However, it could also mean that the work (clients, their needs and concerns), in spite of its many inherent and idiosyncratic properties, is required to fit the established battery of formulae, check-lists, guidelines and competencies. In this outlook, practice does not respond to the inherent meaning of the case. Rather, meaning is imposed on the case according to the skills, resources and interests of the organisation and its practitioners (Howe, 1986). The rise of the manager in social work sees the introduction of a range of skills related largely to defining and measuring performance and outcome. Such an outlook seeks to establish routines, standardised practices and predictable task environments. It is antithetical to depth explanations, professional discretion, creative practice, and tolerance of complexity and uncertainty.

Social work in the market place

If freedom, individuality and personal responsibility are recognised as the human values which drive modernity and best account for its success, their most strident expression remains in the pursuit of a free market economy. The market, based on the rational and self-interested actions of individual men and women, is believed to produce the most efficient, effective and least restrictive social, economic and political systems. During the 1980s, free market principles swept into both the health and the personal social services. The powerful language and philosophy associated with liberal economics does more than set up internal markets, purchasers and providers, clients who are customers, and clients who have the power of choice. It also redefines and gives different meanings to the acts and practices which take place in the name of welfare. When the language used and the conceptual environment it supports undergoes change, the users of that language begin to think and act differently. As language changes so does reality. What social-work practice and clients mean begin to alter in the more bracing climate of neo-liberal economics.

Relationships between social workers and clients change their character from interpersonal to economic, from therapeutic to transactional, from nurturing and supportive to contractual and service-orientated. The relationship becomes a vehicle for market-place dealings. Welfare services become 'commodities' to be traded between those who deliver social-work and those who receive it. The personal relationship, once a central feature of social-work practice and the supposed bedrock of successful support and treatment, is stripped of its social, cultural, emotional and interpersonal dimensions. These are no longer strictly relevant to the client defined as consumer. Practice concentrates on the delivery of material and legal services and the making of performance-orientated decisions and agreements. In this process, welfare services become 'commodified'. The well-being of individuals is more and more reliant on money and markets and not close social relationships. Social ties of support and mutuality are replaced by individualised dealings based on economic transactions. The market becomes the paradigm for all social relationships in which self-reliance, personal enterprise and economic rationalism become the yardsticks by which individuals measure and run their lives.

If the personal relationship between social worker and client is in itself no longer regarded as an essential ingredient of professional practice, training in relationship skills, save for the successful delivery of services, becomes irrelevant and unnecessary. Psychology is not used to help practitioners analyse the causes of client behaviour nor is it used to help the social worker bring about changes in the client. Neither is it used to help practitioners understand the other person and make sense of difficult relationships, including those between worker and client. Knowledge of psychology is used merely to develop those inter-personal skills which facilitate the delivery of the service, the exchange of information and the carrying out of agreed tasks.

THE DISSOLUTION OF SELF AND THE SEARCH FOR PERSONAL MEANING

In a world in which the political pendulum has swung away from the social, the collective and the communal towards the free but isolated individual, the psychological condition and experience of the self also changes. As individuals grasp their essential freedom and discover the thrills as well as the insecurities of autonomy and responsibility, they are wrenched from the comforts as well as constraints of a densely textured communal life underpinned by social expectations and collective responsibilities. If the human self is fundamentally a social self which forms in its relationship with others, the quality of those relationships will influence the kind of self which forms. When freedom becomes the predominant value, the social fabric begins to dissolve. There are intellectual as well as social movements. This can be a time of great creativity, energy and innovation. But the liberated self of the socially disembedded individual, although less confined by the traditions and habits of a close social life, is also a less coherent, more fragmented self. The responsibility is on the individual to make of his or her self what he or she will. But this self is different from the nineteenth-century inner-directed self. Under unrestricted liberal modernism – 'post-modernism' for some – persons are said to exist in a state of continuous self-construction and reconstruction; the self begins to dissolve in a state of permanent self-reflexivity, forming and re-forming across a changing landscape of social relations (Gergen, 1991; Wagner, 1994). This can be exhilarating as well as disturbing. It is the fragmented, disembedded self which corresponds with postmodernity's recognition of the plural and the diverse, the different and the contingent in cultural and political life.

The 'fragmentation of the social body' leads to an increasing concern with security and protection (Eco, cited in Smart, 1993: 31). Although many thrive in this unrestricted, more self-interested world, others feel psychologically diffuse, insecure and uncertain. The anxieties experienced by the insecure and disembedded individual who is charged with the responsibility of making of himself or herself what he or she will in a world which is free, unbounded and competitive, can be debilitating and disruptive. Communitarians argue that the liberal pursuit of securing the conditions for individuals to lead autonomous lives and be free to choose their own values neglects the need for people to feel that they belong. People need to be involved in meaningful communities; they need to be 'socially embedded' because human beings are primarily *social* beings (Bell, 1993). Those who are not embedded in social relationships find it more difficult to realise a coherent sense of self.

The stability of marriages, the rearing of children, the behaviour of adolescents, the morals of the successful and unsuccessful, the caring of others, and the integrity of the psychological self can all be upset in times of heightened anxiety and increased emphasis on the individual. Violence and racial strife increase, more people seek personal counselling in an attempt to give their lives meaning, there is a revival of religious fundamentalism which delivers a social order, a sense of belonging, an ordained certainty and the removal of the anxiety of being responsible for one's own destiny.

THE SOCIAL BASIS OF INDIVIDUALITY

However, when personal and social disturbance threaten to undermine the very interests and freedoms that brought about this dislocation of self, we begin to see a renewal of interest in the psychological and sociological sciences. People begin to ask, once again, why there is so much violence and crime, why the poor are getting relatively poorer, why the patterns of family life are so varied and unstable, and who will care for elderly people and the psychiatrically ill. And when the cry is, 'Something must be done about it', we take the first tentative steps back to collective action based on rational enquiry and the application of the social and psychological sciences to the problems of the individual, society and the relationship between them.

Social-work practices based exclusively on concepts of participation and partnership, political rights and behavioural performance require clients to be rational consumers and responsible agents, encouraged to determine the content of their own futures. However, the impact of the social incoherence generated by the heavy pursuit of neo-liberal values on the integrity of the psychological self makes both social workers and clients capable of non-rational as well as rational behaviour. When people's material worlds are poor and when personal relationships are strained and unsatisfying, levels of stress rise and the emotions drown reason. And when the emotions overrun rational behaviour, when participation, partnership and performance are shattered by impulse, anger and neglect, social-work practice, if it is to cope in a world of disturbed and turbulent relationships, will find itself seeking out psychological and sociological knowledge upon which analytical and inter-personal skills might be based. If the social worker is to make sense of what is going on and respond both sensitively and flexibly, she or he will need more than a repertoire of surface competencies. Social workers will need a theoretical outlook which allows them to make sense of contingent events and non-rational behaviour. They will need knowledge and skills to give them the ability to respond independently and on-the-spot to difficult situations and troubled people.

The tense but unavoidable relationship in modernity between liberty and discipline, justice and welfare, individualism and collectivism is reflected in social work's perennial struggle to define and understand itself. The current swing towards freedom and justice in social work sees a confused eruption in which we find market principles living with ideological pluralism, and the celebration of difference side by side with concerns with what people do rather than with why they do it. Those who believe that social coherence and social embeddedness are related to the development of psychological integrity and social competence will continue to argue that social-work practice needs the insights of psychology and sociology every bit as much as the values of political justice and personal freedom.

Depth explanations do not return social workers to their original starting point. The world of ideas moves on. Modern communitarians are united in their view 'that liberalism does not sufficiently take into account the importance of community for personal identity, moral and political thinking, and judgements about our well-being in the contemporary world . . . liberalism rests on an overly individualistic conception of the self' (Bell, 1993: 4). The social-work theories and practices which square best with communitarian critiques of individual liberalism are those which recognise that the quality of people's social, cultural and material environments has a profound bearing on their psychological development and social competence (Howe, 1995). Personal identities and a sense of belonging form within our relationship history. We are *essentially* social beings. Those psychological and sociological theories which recognise the intimate relationship between the personal and the social are of particular interest to social-workers. Social work practices influenced by perspectives emanating in subject areas such as developmental psychology, attachment theory, cultural psychology and the social formation of the self provide examples which continue to explore traditional social-work ground – the dynamic relationship between the social and the personal. Within such theoretical outlooks might the 'social' be put back into social work.

Chapter 6

Social work, risk and 'the blaming system'

Nigel Parton

Increasingly, social workers and social-welfare agencies are concerned in their day-to-day policies and practices with the issue of risk. Risk assessment, risk management, the monitoring of risk and risk-taking itself have become common activities for both practitioners and managers. Similarly, estimations about risks have become key in identifying priorities and making judgements about the quality of performance and what should be the central focus of professional activities. The purpose of this chapter is to identify some of the areas of social work where notions of risk have taken on a particular significance and to begin the process of analysing what is meant by the term. More fundamentally, however, I want to address why it is the issue has become so important in recent years. My central argument is essentially that risk is not a thing or a set of realities waiting to be unearthed but a way of thinking. As a consequence, social work's increasing obsession(s) with risk(s) point to important changes in both the way social workers think about and constitute their practices and the way social work is itself thought about and thereby constituted more widely.

However, until recently most mainstream social-work texts have had little explicit discussion of risk. As Brearley, in the only book which has centrally addressed the issue for social work, has noted, while 'social work already has a great deal of knowledge and ideas about risk . . . it may not always be expressed in those terms' (1982: 31). Similarly, Alaszewski and Manthorpe (1991: 277) have suggested that, while for commercial institutions such as stock markets, insurance companies and banks the concept of risk is well established and there are clear procedures for measuring and managing risks, there is no equivalent technology within welfare agencies. It seems that it is only recently that the issue has been addressed within mainstream social work in terms of risk. This suggests that an analysis of risk will provide important insights into the changing nature of social work and may encapsulate in important ways the contemporary experiences of what it is to do social work and to be a social worker.

The development of modern social work, particularly in the post-war period, was based on optimistic notions of improvement and rehabilitation and played a small but key element in the growth of 'welfarism'. 'Welfarism' was premised on the wish to encourage social responsibility, the mutuality of social risk and the encouragement of social solidarity and security. The principle of state intervention was made explicit via the institutional framework for maintaining minimum standards. This involved pooling society's resources and spreading the risks across the population and through the life-course. Social insurance summed up the approach and provided the basis for welfare developments in other areas. Persons and activities were to be governed through society, symbolised and coordinated by the state, and based on notions of social citizenship. Professional experts were invested with considerable discretion and trust.

The collapse of 'welfarism' and the growth of neo-liberal critiques have ushered in a quite new situation and one where notions of risk are not simply re-cast but given a much greater significance. No longer is the emphasis on governing through 'society' but through the calculating choices of individuals (Rose, 1993). For neo-liberalism the political subject is less a social citizen with powers and obligations deriving from membership of a collective body than an individual whose citizenship is active. It is an individualised conception of citizenship where the emphasis is upon personal fulfilment and individual responsibility. At the same time, the impact of global market forces has hastened dislocation in most areas of economic and social life, reinforcing a whole variety of insecurities, uncertainties and fears. Not only can changes in social work be seen to reflect these wider and rapid social and economic transformations but also the nature of social work is such that it is intimately implicated and involved. The growing concerns about risk in social work can thus be understood as both reflecting these increased anxieties, uncertainties and insecurities and as providing a rationale for coping, understanding and responding to the new situation. For while there is growing concern that certain sections of the population are increasingly marginalised and vulnerable, there is also a greater emphasis on professional responsibility and accountability for the safety and well-being of those they come into contact with. Concerns about risk can be seen to articulate and represent these tensions and contradictions most clearly.

RISK AND SOCIAL WORK

The area of social work where the issue of risk has been seen as most crucial is that of child protection and child welfare more generally. In effect, the development of official policy and guidance in recent years has been concerned with the refinement of practices, systems and knowledge whereby 'high risk' can be identified (DoH, 1988; DoH, 1991a).

Until 1987, much of the public criticism directed at practitioners and fuelled by the public enquiries and the media (DHSS, 1982; DoH, 1991a) was that child deaths occurred, in major part, because practitioners failed to identify and act upon the key factors associated with child abuse and thereby unnecessarily put children at high risk. If only social workers and other professionals had familiarised themselves with the 'known characteristics of child abuse' and integrated them into their everyday practice, tragedies could be avoided. The approach was exemplified by the Beckford Report (London Borough of Brent, 1985; Parton, 1986), which argued that: 'society should sanction, in "high risk" cases, the removal of such children for an appreciable time' (p. 289).

Following the Cleveland affair and subsequent inquiry (Secretary of State for Social Services, 1988), the focus of concern shifted to the powers of welfare professionals to intervene into the private family and remove children unwarrantably. However, the net effect was to underline the importance of trying to identify and assess 'high-risk' even further. For in theory, the identification of the actually or potentially 'high risk' case or situation provides the mechanism for ensuring that children are protected, unwarrantable interventions can be avoided and scarce resources are allocated efficiently. While it is now recognised that the identification of risk using a positivist scientific approach, as suggested by the Beckford Report and earlier disease-model approaches, is inappropriate (see Parton, 1989; Dingwall, 1989), the need to identify high risk lies at the core of what constitutes the nature of contemporary child protection policy and practice. The Department of Health guide (1988), *Protecting Children*, addresses the key issue of whether a family is considered safe for a child, whether it can be made safe or whether it is so potentially dangerous that alternatives have to be found. While the guide accepts that child protection work can never be risk free, it is explicitly concerned with trying to address the assessment of risk and hence the improvement of decision-making and thereby would 'provide opportunities for more effective supervision and management of the social work task' (DoH, 1988: 3). In effect, the guide attempts to provide a map whereby practitioners can organise and classify information for the purposes of assessing and making decisions. The social assessment is seen as strategic in allocating cases to their correct category and thereby coordinating resources and expertise. Professional judgement and decision-making is essentially concerned with the identification and assessment of 'high risk'.

These issues are embedded in the Social Services Inspectorate framework for *Evaluating Performance in Child Protection* (1993). For example, in two of the four criteria used for evaluating the first common standard, that 'in each child protection case, all staff ensure that the welfare of the child is paramount', risk is key:

- the child is provided with immediate protection in situations where their life is *at risk* or there is a likelihood of sustaining a serious injury if this action is not taken;
- in situations where there are child protection concerns, but the child is not in a life-threatening situation or *at risk* of serious injury or harm, careful consideration is given to the *degree of risk*, how best to protect the child and to timescales for planned monitoring at an initial investigation being carried out.

(1993: 14–15, my emphasis)

The notions of risk, harm and protection are clearly inter-related. However, it is also clear that the way risk is understood, applied and operated in everyday practice is at a very poor level of development. For example, in an evaluation of child protection procedures in four area child protection committee areas (Giller *et al.*, 1992), it was concluded that although risk analysis was said to be a central part of each case conference, in none of the areas examined did the procedures address what risk analysis might involve and how professionals should approach it. Similarly, the Audit Commission (1994) has noted that much field social-work time is used in carrying out inappropriate child protection investigations. They recommend that risk indicators should be developed that trigger a full investigation and that the Department of Health and the Welsh Office develop guidance on risk management.

In other areas of social work the concern with risk has similarly grown. For example, the role of the Probation Service has shifted from being primarily concerned with the assessment and management of need to the assessment and management of risk (ACOP, 1994). This shift has been prompted by a number of administrative and legislative changes, notably the Audit Commission Report (1989), the Criminal Justice Act 1991 and the Statement of National Objectives (1993). For example, the Audit Report (1989) argued that probation had already changed its focus from social casework to the more pragmatic role of dealing with high-risk offenders. The Report argued that the Probation Service should concentrate its efforts on developing more stringent forms of community supervision, and intensive probation programmes, so that the courts might be persuaded to use non-custodial options in the sentencing of high-risk offender groups (such as recidivist burglars and thieves) who would otherwise be given a prison sentence. The Probation Service should concentrate on its core functions of court work and the policing of supervision orders. The traditional social-work aspects of the work were not a priority and should be carried out by a less-skilled voluntary sector.

The area of mental health, particularly in relation to the mentally disordered offender, over the last twenty years has been dominated by debates about the concept of high risk. Repeatedly, attempts have been made to single out a group of worrying offenders and permit special protective sentences for them. Considerable debate has taken place in terms of whether it is possible to predict high risk and the civil liberties issues involved (Floud and Young, 1981; Prins, 1986; and Wood, 1988). While the Reed Committee Report (1992) emphasises the need for community care over custodial institutional care and the importance of providing care and treatment by health and personal social services, the need to identify those who are dangerous or high-risk cases is seen as important if the balance of service provision and care and control is to be maintained and perhaps refined (Zito Trust, 1995).

Within the general area of community care, however, the notion of risk seems much less central. While there is literature on risk and older people (Brearley, 1982), it is really only in relation to elder abuse (Social Services Inspectorate, 1992) that the issue is seen as central (Swanhunter, 1994). The official and professional language of community care is in terms of the assessment and management of 'need' rather than 'risk' (Stevenson and Parsloe, 1993). What seems likely, however, is that as concern about elder abuse develops in a context of a growing number of older people in the population and where more and more emphasis is placed upon maintaining people in their own home, the focus for assessment, decision-making and the allocation of scarce resources may be framed much more explicitly in terms of risk.

Perhaps the most explicit evidence of the increased concern and centrality of risk for social-work and welfare agencies is the development of the Risk Initiative by the Social Services Inspectorate (SSI). The overall project is intended to provide a link between SSI core inspections during the 1994/95 work programme by developing the common theme of 'risk' within each of them. It starts from the premise that the personal social services are concerned primarily with risks to service-users, carers and care workers, and the impact on this of the policies and actions of assessors, care managers, care workers, managers and agencies. A number of 'risk' standards have been developed for inspections. They have been designed not to add significant elements to inspections but to highlight and pull together material relating to risk issues which are already gathered in other ways. Inspectors are asked to apply a number of standards: (1) whether senior managers ensure that there are policies, procedures and guidance on risk issues, that these are understood and followed by staff of the Social Services Department and other service providers, and that they are regularly reviewed; (2) that risks are analysed and appropriately managed at all stages of the referral, assessment and care management process; (3) that the suitability of prospective staff members (and other people providing care such as foster parents) is thoroughly checked before appointment, and when staff are in post they receive appropriate guidance, training and support to enable them to perform tasks with awareness and understanding of possible risk issues; and (4) that senior staff and care workers receive appropriate equipment, guidance, training and support in relation to issues of health, safety and security of users, staff and premises. More than ever it seems that the quality of agency policy and professional practice will be judged in terms of the way they prioritise, assess, plan and respond to risk.

At one level this emphasis on risk can be understood in terms of the changing political and social climate in which social work now operates. No longer can social work operate behind a paternalistic benevolent cloak, for users are expected to be given increased choice and autonomy and in a context where they must take more responsibility for their actions. Community alternatives are being developed in all spheres so that institutional provision is reserved for the few who may be a danger to themselves or to others. Need is increasing as a consequence of widening inequalities (Goodman and Webb, 1994; Wilkinson, 1994), changing demography and increasing expectations but in a context where welfare resources are not expanding and in many areas are reducing. Risk has become the key criterion for targeting scarce resources, protecting the most vulnerable and making professionals and agencies accountable.

Tony Bottoms (1977) was perhaps the first person in this country to note the significance of the increased official interest in the idea of dangerousness (Campbell, 1995) or 'high risk' in his analysis of changes in relation to penal policy in the 1970s. This interest coincided with the growing tendency to advocate or impose more severe penalties for offenders regarded as 'really serious', while advocating a reduction in penalties for the ordinary or run-of-the-mill offender. The use of long sentences *increased* in a period when there was a general *decrease* in sentence severity – what Bottoms called '*bifurcation*'. For bifurcation to become a reality, one has to *believe* in the possibility of separating the high risk from the rest and have the expertise and systems in place to carry that through. The assessment and management of actual or potential high risk becomes the central concern and activity. In all the areas where social work operates where there is an increased emphasis upon keeping people in the community, where resources are limited and where the costs of getting things wrong are considerable, the 'high risk' criterion seems to offer an objective yardstick for deciding who is safe to be let out. It has become the key focus in modern classification systems for the purposes of allocating people to different forms of social regulation. Whereas it used to be 'moral character', and sometimes was 'treatability', increasingly it tends to be 'high risk' (Cohen, 1994; Feeley and Simon, 1994).

THE NATURE OF RISK

Having outlined the areas of social work where risk seems to have become an area of increasing concern over recent years and offering some initial analysis as to why this might be the case, I now want to begin the process of unpacking what is meant by risk. The concept originally emerged in the seventeenth century in the context of gambling. For this purpose a specialised mathematical analysis of chance was developed. Risk then meant the probability of an event occurring, combined with the magnitude of the losses or gains entailed (Hacking, 1975). Subsequently the analysis of probabilities became the basis of scientific knowledge, transforming the nature of evidence, of knowledge, of authority and logic. Any process or activity had its probabilities of success or failures. In the eighteenth century the analysis of risk had important uses in marine insurance. The chances of a ship coming safely home were set against the chances of it being lost at sea. The idea of risk was neutral and simply took account of the probability of gains and losses. The calculation of risk became deeply entrenched in science and manufacturing as a theoretical base for decision-making. In the process, notions of probability became embedded in modern ways of thinking.

However, as Mary Douglas (1986, 1992) has argued, as notions of risk have become more central to politics and public policy its connection with technical calculations of probability has weakened. While it continues to combine a probabilistic measure of the occurrence of the primary event(s) with a measure of the consequences of those events, the concept of risk is now only associated with negative outcomes. Definitions of risk are now only associated with notions of hazard, danger, exposure, harm and loss. For example, the Royal Society Study Group recently defined 'risk' 'as the probability that a particular adverse event occurs during a stated period of time, or results from a particular challenge' (Report of a Royal Society Study Group, 1992: 2). The risk that is the central concept for policy debates has now not got much to do with neutral probability calculations. 'The original connection is only indicated by arm-waving in the direction of possible science: the word *risk* now means danger; *high risk* means a lot of danger' (Douglas, 1992: 24, original emphasis).

Whereas originally a high risk meant a game in which a throw of the die had a strong probability of bringing great pain or great loss, risk now only refers to negative outcomes. The word now only means bad risks. The language of risk is reserved for talk of undesirable outcomes. Whereas previously 'danger' would have been the right word, '*danger* does not have the aura of science or afford the pretension of a possible precise calculation' (Douglas, 1992: 25, original emphasis). The language of danger having turned into the language of risk thus gives the impression of being calculable and scientific. But this is not simply about linguistic style. The possibility of a scientifically objective decision about exposure to danger is part of the new complex of ideas. Not only is risk superficially scientific, it is also future-orientated and predictive. It looks forward to assess the dangers ahead.

However, Douglas argues that while this is an important shift it is not the major significance of the contemporary emphasis on risk. 'The big difference is not in the predictive uses of risk, but in its forensic functions' (1992: 27). The concept of risk emerges as a key idea for contemporary times because of its uses as a forensic resource. The more culturally individualised a society becomes, the more significant becomes the forensic potential of the idea of risk. Its forensic uses are particularly important in the development of different types of blaming system, and 'the one we are in now is almost ready to treat every death as chargeable to someone's account, every accident as caused by someone's criminal negligence, every sickness a threatened prosecution' (1992: 15–16).

Douglas sees the contemporary concerns with risk as fulfilling a similar role to that previously played by 'sin' in earlier times but the emphasis and implications are quite different. Previously, disasters were explained in terms of sins. However, whereas risks are future-orientated, sins are backward-looking: first the disaster, then the explanation of its cause in an earlier transgression. There is, however, another important difference. To be 'at risk' is equivalent to being sinned against, being vulnerable to the events caused by others, whereas being 'in sin' means being the cause of harm. The rhetoric of sin used to uphold the community, vulnerable to the misbehaviour of the individual, while the rhetoric of risk upholds the individual who is seen as *vulnerable* to the behaviour of the community, bureaucrats or powerful experts. While sin acts to protect the *community* from vulnerability risk acts to protect the *individual* from vulnerability. It has come to play a key role in the contemporary blaming system.

THE RISK SOCIETY

For much of the post-war period there was a general mood of optimism that science and technology, together with the activities of the welfare state, had generally ushered in a period of prosperity and permanent improvement. There was an enthusiasm and support for experts and professionals. Science had made things different and better for everyone. As a result it was believed we were able to recognise real danger, the causes of which could be objectively identified, backed by the authority of research and theory. Chance and mystery had been reduced to the margins not yet claimed by science. But generally it was believed that, because of our objective, accurate knowledge of the world and our powerful technologies, our blaming behaviour was capable of going direct to real causes. Real blaming was possible because of its objective basis in scientific knowledge. It was assumed that human order by the development and application of science could be subject to human control so that things could be regular, repeatable and predictable. Notions of reason and rationality informed the development of a blaming system that was increasingly positivistic, and believed that not only could causes be objectively identified but that they could be subject to improvement and change.

Increasingly, however, contemporary society has become characterised by widespread scepticism about providential reason – the idea that increased secular understanding of the world leads to a safer and more rewarding existence. There is a growing recognition that science and modern technologies are double-edged, creating new harms and negative consequences as well as offering beneficial possibilities.

The issue of child abuse provides a key exemplar of these important shifts. During the 1950s and 1960s research and theorising about child abuse assumed it was a reality which had been hidden in the privacy of the family and hence hidden from public and professional view. Science, particularly medical science, was seen as important for establishing the reliable foundations for our knowledge of child abuse and hence informing policy and practice. What was needed was research to rip away the layers of disguise and uncover the underlying reality. The development of science and research would allow professionals to identify abuse and intervene benignly on behalf of children. The model was based on what I have called elsewhere (Parton, 1985) the disease model of child abuse and developed from the approach articulated by Henry Kempe and his colleagues (1962) in Denver in terms of the 'battered child syndrome'. The use of a number of clinical technologies, particularly the X-ray, proved crucial not only in discovering otherwise hidden signs and symptoms, but also in informing the way the problem was thought about, diagnosed and treated, essentially as a medical entity, for many years to come. While by the late 1970s the term 'child abuse' referred to a wide variety of situations that varied in form and degree, the 'battered child syndrome' remained the root metaphor.

By the mid-1980s, however, a number of critiques had developed which severely questioned the empirical and conceptual basis for such an approach – see Parton (1989) for a summary. It was recognised that much of the scientific and clinical research was not nearly as neutral as was assumed and that as a consequence there were a number of unforeseen and unintended consequences in the dominant approach to policy and practice. In particular, it was argued that as a result some children were continuing to suffer and die while others were inappropriately identified and in danger as a result of the problems of false negative and false positive predictions. The positivist scientific approach was found fundamentally wanting. These issues were very publicly played out via the Cleveland inquiry and subsequently in Rochdale, Orkney and elsewhere. One of the messages to emerge was that the system which had been set up to identify, regulate and police child abuse was itself culpable. The scientific basis to the way we had attempted to tackle child abuse seemed to have as many negative consequences for children, families and professionals as it did positives. Dennis Howitt has argued that science played an important role in what have been seen as errors in child abuse work:

> the close interplay between the 'science' of child abuse and practice is important to understanding how some sorts of child abuse error occur. It is the incorporation of key elements of positivist science into social policy. This mode of thinking, to the extent to which it occurs in the thinking of all professionals involved in dealing with child abuses, is part of the genesis of errors.
>
> (1992: 49)

Although different in the detail of their manifestation, most areas of professional practice and decision-making, and the research and scientific basis on which they are practised, have come in for similar criticism over recent years. As a consequence of the pace and form(s) of change, many of our assumptions concerning the notion of state, science, expertise and knowledge have been subject to increasing doubt, scepticism and uncertainty. To live in the world increasingly has the feeling of riding a 'juggernaut' (Giddens, 1990). No aspect of our activities follows a predestined course, and all are open to contingency.

Ulrich Beck (1992a, 1992b) characterises contemporary society as a 'risk society'. This does not simply refer to the fact that contemporary social life introduces new forms of danger for humanity but that living in the risk society means living with a calculative attitude to the open possibilities of action with which we are continually confronted. In circumstances of increasing uncertainty and apparent doubt the notion of risk has a particular purchase.

In the shift from the modern society to the risk society, the quality and nature of communal concerns and values shift. According to Beck, in the former the focal concerns are with substantive and positive goals of social change, attaining something good and trying to ensure that everyone has a stake and a fair share. However, in the risk society the normative basis is safety and the Utopia is peculiarly negative and defensive – preventing the worst and protection from harm. As a result statements on risk become the 'moral statements' of society (Beck, 1992a: 176). The axial principle is the distribution not of goods but of bads – the distribution of hazards, dangers and risks.

The concept of risk becomes fundamental to the way both lay actors and experts experience and organise the social world. Risk assessment and management are crucial to the colonisation, understanding and control of the future, but at the same time necessarily open up the unknown. Risk assessment suggests precision, and even quantification, but by its nature is imperfect. Given the mobile character of the social world and the mutable and controversial nature of abstract systems of knowledge, most forms of assessment contain numerous imponderables. This issue – the central yet uncertain nature of risk and risk assessment – is key to understanding the changing nature and role of science and knowledge and hence experts in contemporary society (Luhmann, 1993).

The risk society is thus also a self-critical, reflexive society. Risks come into being where traditions and assumed values have deteriorated. Determinations of risk straddle the distinction between objective and value dimensions. Moral standards are not asserted openly but in quantitative, theoretical and causal forms. But notions of risk are never settled and are continually moving. 'The concept of risk is like a probe which permits us over and over again to investigate the entire construction plan, as well as every individual speck of cement in the structure of civilization for potentials of self-endangerment' (Beck, 1992a: 176). Risk becomes central in a society which is taking leave of the past but which is also opening itself up to a problematic future. Risk becomes closely inter-related with reflexivity. For to assess risk in contemporary society requires the process of 'reflexive scientization' (Beck, 1992a) or 'reflexivity' (Giddens, 1990, 1991) in what we do and the way we do it, both individually and institutionally. The 'reflexive monitoring of risk is intrinsic to institutionalised risk systems' (Giddens, 1991: 119).

Beck differentiates between 'reflexive scientization' and what went before, 'primary scientization'. The model of primary scientisation is based on the 'naïveté' that the methodical scepticism of science can be institutionalised but reserved to the *objects* of science and not to itself. However, scientific methods and pronouncements carry within themselves the standards for their own critique and possible abolition. Scientific developments undermine their own foundations through the continuity of their own success. 'In the course of the *triumph* and generalization of the norms of scientific argument, a completely different situation arises' (Beck, 1992a: 164–5, original emphasis). This unbinding of scepticism lies at the heart of the conditions of reflexive scientisation. While scientific, and professional, dogma is undermined, its original authority and foundations themselves become increasingly uncertain and shaky. So while science becomes indispensable in the risk society it also becomes devoid of its original validity claims. Science thus experiences a loss of security and confidence in both its internal and external relations and hence a decline in its power. This results in increased conflict between experts and lay people. Beck suggests that one good indicator of this is the increase in 'medical malpractice' lawsuits, but others would include the increased need for and use of complaints procedures in social work of one sort or another.

However, while science is becoming human and is packed with errors and mistakes and divergent interpretations, the risk society cannot do without it either. The recourse to scientific analysis and results for the socially binding definition of truth and decision-making becomes more and more necessary but less and less sufficient. As a result of this growing disparity between the necessary and sufficient conditions of truth, the number and range of grey areas open to dispute grows. 'The target groups and users of scientific results become more dependent on scientific arguments in *general*, but at the same time more independent of *individual* findings and the judgment of science regarding the truth and reality of its statements' (Beck, 1992a: 167, original emphasis).

Risk and science are very dependent on each other in the

contemporary situation. Whereas previously hazards and dangers were directly perceptible to the senses – particularly the nose and the eyes – the ways risks are thought about almost escape perception. Because something assaults our senses does not mean it is a risk. Risks in effect only exist in the formulae, theorems or assessments which construct them. They remain invisible and are based on causal interpretations and predictions and thus exist in terms of the knowledge about them. We are dealing with a theoretical and hence a scientised consciousness, even in the everyday consciousness of risk. They must always be imagined, implied and ultimately believed. The suggested causality always remains more or less uncertain and tentative. Risks can thus be changed, magnified or minimised within the knowledge of them and to that extent they are particularly open to social definition and social construction. The mass media and the scientific and legal professions thus play key political roles in the defining, re-defining and constitution of risks.

It is in this respect that it becomes evident that contemporary concerns with risk reflect ways of organising and thinking about the world rather than refer to some external or hidden reality. Thus while a significant part of expert thinking and public discourse is about risk profiling – analysing what, in the current state of knowledge and in current conditions, is the distribution of risks in the given milieu of action – such profiles are subject to continual critique and revision. No longer does expert knowledge create stable inductive arenas, for it is liable to produce unintended or unforeseen consequences or its findings may be open to diverse interpretations. The self and the wider institutional arrangements have to be continually assessed, monitored and reviewed and thereby reflexively made. Nothing can be taken for granted. So although science has become indispensable to this process, it is incapable of truth. 'Where science used to be convincing *qua* science, today, in view of the contradictory babble of scientific tongues, the *faith* in science or the *faith* in alternative science (or *this* method, *this* approach, *this* orientation) becomes decisive' (Beck, 1992a: 169, original emphasis). Under conditions of reflexive scientisation, the production or mobilisation of belief becomes a central source for the social enforcement of validity claims.

Thus the emergence of the risk society arises because of the undermining and loss of faith concerning science, knowledge and various hierarchies of truth and power. However, rather than replace these emerging doubts and uncertainties with new certainties, the process continues amidst growing complexities and scepticism such that reflexivity and calculative attitudes to the future become more pervasive. It is not by chance, then, that the increased focus on risk in social work has coincided with the decline in trust in social workers' expertise and decision-making, and the growing reliance on increasingly complex systems of audit, monitoring and quality controls (see the chapter by John Clarke in this volume). For audit has become central for responding to the pluralities of expertise and the inherent controversy and undecidability of their truth claims. As we have already noted, the key contemporary significance of risk is in its forensic functions and the importance this has for making experts accountable – justifying what they do and why they do it.

In recent years social-work practitioners and their managers have been subject to a range of new techniques for exercising critical scrutiny over their practice often formulated in budgetary and accountancy terms. What I am suggesting is that the emphasis on risk has also contributed to this increased role of auditing – in the widest sense – to which social work is both subject and in which it plays an active part. Whereas the trust in science, technology and experts – social workers – has been undermined, audit has increased, and this process is intimately related to our pervasive concerns about risk (Rose, 1993) which plays a key role in the 'blaming system' and new forms of accountability.

As Michael Power (1994a, 1994b) has argued, audit in a range of different forms has come to replace the trust once accorded to professionals both by their clients – now users and customers – and the authorities which employ, legitimate and constitute them. The constant demands for audit both gives expression to and contributes to the erosion of trust, and the expertise and positive knowledge of human conduct on which it was based. As we have seen, such audits and inspections increasingly use notions of risk – the assessment of, management of, procedures for – in order to judge the quality of the practices that are being investigated whether this be the individual case or more generally in the organisational processes of welfare agencies themselves. What is particularly worrying is that where concerns about danger, hazards and risks become all-pervasive they can assume a permanent institutional form – and there is evidence to suggest that this is happening. It is as if a state of emergency is being introduced in order to cope with the growing risk but which is itself a way of thinking and is socially constructed. Responding to risk becomes the norm. It gives birth to a language that crawls with expressions like 'control', 'official approval', 'management responsibility' and so on. In short, the pervasiveness of risk in a context where the trust in science and experts is replaced by audit can lead to new forms of organisational defensiveness and authoritarianism. It is as if once concerns about risk become all-pervasive the requirement to develop and follow organisational procedures becomes dominant and the room for professional manoeuvre and creativity is severely limited. Ironically, once risk becomes institutionalised the ability and willingness of professionals to take risks – in the original sense of possible positive as well as negative outcomes – is curtailed.

CONCLUSION

In this chapter I have argued that our increasing obsession with risk can be seen to reflect the new vulnerabilities and new anxieties arising from various global changes and our attempts to respond to these. The neutral vocabulary of risk attempts to provide a bridge between the known 'facts' and experiences of existence and the construction of a new moral community. It aspires to provide a generalised mechanism whereby the needs of welfare and the needs of justice can be met. As Douglas has argued:

> the idea of risk could have been custom-made. Its universalizing terminology, its abstractness, its power of condensation, its scientificity, its connection with objective analysis, make it perfect. Above all, its forensic uses fit the tool to the task of building a culture that supports a modern industrial society.
>
> (1992: 15)

Notions of risk have thus become central in a culture which needs a common forensic vocabulary with which to hold individuals accountable. Yet disputes about risk have become endemic and self-generating. Every institution is increasingly aware of its liability for exposing employees and customers/users to risk so that everything has to be spelled out in order to cover for any future negative consequences. In the process of protecting against one category of risk it may be that people are exposed to another.

Thus risk has unequivocally come to mean danger from future damage. However, the nature and gravity of any risk has become a matter for the ascribed experts to determine and their judgements may vary and be in dispute. Crucially, however, it has to be assumed

that the matter is ascertainable otherwise its rationale for accountability weakens. These issues have gathered in significance as our
experiences and awareness of uncertainty and doubt have increased
in recent times. Risk has come to play a key role in the contemporary
blaming system both in and of social work more generally.

ACKNOWLEDGEMENTS

I would like to thank Hazel Kemshall, Mike Walsh, Jan Waterson,
Bill Jordan and Corinne Wattam for the various discussions we have
had related to risk and social work. I hope they feel this chapter
benefited as a result.

Chapter 7

Telling tales

Probation in the contemporary social formation

Robert Harris

PROLEGOMENON: THE PROBATION OFFICER AS STORYTELLER

> All in all, postmodernity can be seen as restoring to the world what modernity, presumptuously, had taken away; as a re-enchantment of the world that modernity tried hard to dis-enchant. It is the modern artifice that has been dismantled; the modern conceit of meaning-legislating reason that has been exposed, condemned and put to shame. It is that artifice and that reason, the reason of the artifice, that stands accused in the court of postmodernity
>
> (Bauman, 1992: x).

This chapter is an essay on what we may loosely term 'the postmodern condition of probation'. That it is both simplified and truncated results not only from limitations imposed by form (one chapter in a book about contemporary applied social science and social work) or authorial ability (severely circumscribed though that doubtless is) but, more significantly, from two theoretical considerations. First, in the postmodern world *any* writer's 'authority' is questionable and liable to be impugned and undermined. The 'author' becomes – in both senses of the word – a partial narrator, a mere collector even of the thoughts and writings of others, yielding a text which it is for the reader to create and re-create in multitudinous ways (very different perspectives are thrown on this point by Booth, 1961; Barthes, 1977; Eco, 1979; Genette, 1980; Docherty, 1987).

Second, by definition no account of the postmodern condition can be complete. This limitation, however, is inevitably vulnerable to conscription to the cause of *a priori* excuse for analytic inadequacy – a 'postmodernist cop-out' – and it is for the reader to determine whether this text stands convicted of this heresy. For a paper about professional action to be so convicted would be condemnation indeed, of course, and in anticipation of such a charge it is worth pointing out that there is in the postmodern perspective, guided no doubt by the revisionist hermeneutics of Gadamer in particular (Gadamer, 1975), an increasing fusion between performance and narration, interpretation and reality. Hence interpretation comes to be constituted as a form of action, shifting the tradition of which it is a part, so contributing to contemporary perceptions of reality. This is certainly not a case of art imitating life or even life imitating art, but of life and art becoming almost indistinguishable. Never, for example, have social and literary theory been so proximal. This point defines a theoretical piece such as this as being itself a form of intervention.

The point is relevant also for the Probation Service, whose location in the contemporary social formation oddly straddles the modern and the postmodern. The political discourse which, with varying degrees of enthusiasm, probation embraces is decidedly modernist: it entails an expectation that contemporary problems of crime and criminal justice can be solved in a manner appropriate to the laboratory experiment. The evaluation of probation's effectiveness is therefore tailored less to professional than to political imperatives; and the modes of managerialist inspection to which it is (in common with many other professions) subject charge the service with imposing rationality and order on a world which appears inexplicably devoid of structure or purpose. Yet probation's capacity to manufacture these desirable products – less crime, the effective control of its charges during that great bulk of time when they are not under direct and effective surveillance – is very limited. The worlds of probation politics and probation practice can seldom have been further apart, and the Probation Service is in need of a new and different mode of self-comprehension.

This is by no means to recommend a repudiation of contemporary politics, however, for little could be more important than for the service to seize the opportunities which current political conjunctions have opened up for it. What is required is not substitution but augmentation, a professional perspective standing in dialectical relation to the political one, each offering a critical perspective on the other. It is important to remember that history did not stop yesterday, and that just as yesterday's truism is today's anachronism, so will much of what is professed and practised today be viewed with incredulity by generations still to come. Today's reality constitutes only a frozen moment in an unfolding world, and it would be helpful were the service to initiate a thoughtful debate – not a private one among the *cognoscenti* but one which embraces those outside its internal discourse – on its aims and ambitions, and on the nature and potential of its role in criminal justice.

This chapter's modest and partial contribution to this process is to invite the service to engage once again with its narrative self, and to render it appropriate to the contemporary world. In probation's understandable rush to embrace the modernist political discourse it has abandoned those parts of its own tradition which enable it to appeal to other audiences, or to the same audience in a different way. This chapter sets the scene for such an engagement, but it *does* only set the scene, and is not definitive.

The Probation Service underwent a transformation around 1967–72, during which period it changed from a pre-modern to a modern organisation. To simplify but not caricature, prior to the early 1970s the Probation Service was a small, friendly, homogeneous community with a relatively simple range of tasks which it undertook in a spirit of kindness and good humour. Even allowing for the dangers of golden age theorising there is plausibility in the recollections of retired officers who speak (significantly for our purposes) of the pre-1970s service as a 'big village' in which training (then a Home Office responsibility) was a shared experience; when everyone knew everyone else – or could at least identify with ease mutual acquaintances when a stranger officer was encountered; when relations with courts were personal, close and based on mutual respect; and when there was homogeneity of purpose and value which helped officers define themselves as members of a coherent and organic, albeit geographically dispersed, community.

During this period a consonance of purpose manifested itself more publicly too, in a way which enabled a particular image of the service to be presented in popular form through television and literature. Probation and court are dramatic settings full of human interest and with strong narrative possibilities, and their public face was once regularly portrayed in narrative form. There were autobiographical snippets (for example, Dark, 1939; Watson, 1939, 1969; Henriques, 1950; Cooks, 1958;[1] Todd, 1963, 1964[2]), case-books (Le Mesurier, 1931; Reakes, 1953), journalistic observations (St John, 1961), and numerous moral tales of reformed criminals, some revealing how their lives and behaviour had been transformed by a chance given by someone who trusted them, others how their lives had been ruined by the degradation of prison (for example, Benney, 1936, 1948; McCartney, 1939; Maxwell, 1956; Slater, 1967).

Though (or perhaps because) they were often sentimentalised and didactic, such books and the sad or humorous tales they told had an immediacy of impact on a public audience which is today largely dependent for its images of crime and criminals on the punitive stereotypes of government pronouncement and tabloid press. Yet in their observational, reporting, recording and interventive activities probation officers are story-tellers *par excellence*, offering up for the consumption of other professionals not 'the truth' *tout court* but a rendition of it which will be comprehensible and acceptable both in the language of their own 'invisible' trade (Pithouse, 1987) and in that of their intended audience. But probation officers are not 'mere' narrators standing aloof from the action, commenting, interpreting and advising in dispassionate terms. On the contrary, their narratives have about them a tactical aesthetic designed to promote a humane response from their audience, and even to inculcate a set of socio-political ideas by insinuating speculative but plausible social explanations of a specific criminal act into a quasi-legal document. This is narrative as action indeed.

The Probation Service has a second striking characteristic which also constitutes part of the theme of this chapter: its *marginality*. Probation is marginal as a profession and marginal to criminal justice, social work and both central and local government. It claims a libertarian and egalitarian value base but daily imposes control on its charges, not so much by its daily interactions with them (which are doubtless overwhelmingly well-meaning and supportive), but by its very existence, and in particular by the suspensiveness of its power (Harris and Webb, 1987). Given the socio-political status of the Probation Service, it would be a naïve offender who did not regard the probation office as an antechamber to a less pleasant locus for punishment; yet this gloomy perception is only half the truth, for the probation office is simultaneously a place of warmth, support and confession.

In addition, the Probation Service deals with many people who are themselves marginal, not only socially and economically but as both law-abiding citizens and criminals: if probationers were unambiguously law-abiding they would not come the way of the service; unambiguously criminal, and they would be in prison with the 'big-timers'. For all the attempts of government to clarify probation's role and functions its work remains, for the time being at least, a case study in the translation of equivocation into practice, a daily reminder of the problem of action in a world where, while the problems which arise outnumber the solutions available to solve them, such a state of affairs is politically impossible to acknowledge.

It is often from the margins that critique most powerfully comes, but from a position of marginal involvement, not of exclusion. In literature, for example, the contributions of work from the margins – rediscovered women writers, black writers and writers of new literatures in English – have been among the most significant of the last decade, the critique of mainstream literary culture which they both present and represent being the more powerful because it emerges from the cracks of the mainstream activity. So it is with probation: an activity both marginal and intellectual is well placed to offer a critique of the mainstream, but once its marginality is abandoned or confiscated critique becomes more difficult. For not only is self-critique tactically difficult in a hostile political climate but, more subtly, viewed from the mainstream the world itself genuinely looks different.

The Probation Service regularly encounters situations in which competing explanations of human behaviour inconsiderately emerge, explanations which demand simultaneous genuflections at the altars of freedom and determinism. Who after all can deny that existential moment when a choice must be made as to whether or not to commit a crime? Equally, who can doubt that these matters are not randomly distributed, that were the middle classes to begin experiencing centuries of discrimination, dislocation and disadvantage the numbers of middle-class criminals would steadily, if inexplicably in individual terms, increase? Or that their modes of deviance would come to be regarded with more than passing disfavour by those in charge of the new social order? Whether by chance or design the traditional ambiguities of probation conveniently address the ambiguities which arise from ontological uncertainties of this kind, uncertainties experienced no less sharply by sentencers than by probation officers. The ambiguities of probation ease the administration of justice in an unjust world.

This chapter examines aspects of these forms of marginality. In doing so, it will show that probation's marginality has greatly diminished as the service has been moved centre-stage by a government anxious to impose order and reason throughout the social world. In this, of course, the service is being dealt with no differently from other public services and utilities (Harris, 1994): the processes of centralising policy but devolving administrative responsibility for delivering it, imposing tight financial controls and accountability, injecting competition in a mixed supply economy, emphasising efficiency and effectiveness (Home Office, 1987) and measuring value for money are common elements of current public-sector management strategy. In fact the Probation Service, which at the end of the 1980s retained much the form and structure of ten years earlier, was remarkably sheltered from the restructuring experienced in the fields of health, education and the public utilities.

BEFORE THE 1970s: PRE-MODERN PROBATION

It is not strange that Jim, with all his time unhappily on his hands and the call of the young in his ears, answers the whistle of the boys in the street, 'bad lads' though his mother calls them, and in his heart he knows them to be. It is more tolerable than staying in the little overcrowded home, where mother is cross, and baby crying, and father down on him because he hasn't a job. . . . Neither was he a bad lad by nature: he made a good impression and showed no vicious propensities. Some pleasing traits came out in the home account of him: his fondness for the little ones, and for animals, – the fact that when in work he gave his mother all his wages and was well content with the few shillings pocket-money she allowed him. But he lacked training; the parental control was weak and intermittent, and his own ideas of right and wrong had got very dim during the last months of unemployment and evil company. In short he was going down-hill. Unless pulled up in time, not all his good natural qualities would save him from becoming an habitual criminal.

(Le Mesurier, 1931: 57–61)

. . . understanding itself is not to be thought of so much as an action of one's subjectivity but as the placing of oneself within a process of tradition, in which past and present are constantly fused.

(Gadamer, 1975: 258)

Probation has, over the century or so of its existence as a recognisable entity, been transformed from a small agency, responsible for doing good at the fringes of the criminal justice system, to a fairly large organisation, complex in purpose and structure, responsible for delivering non-custodial and post-custodial community corrections.

The modern era of probation began between about 1967 (when it assumed responsibility for parole supervision) and 1972 (when the Criminal Justice Act extended its activities). From then on successive governments have sought to define the service as an arm of the criminal justice and penal systems complementary to the police and prison services, and to play down those 'softer' activities conventionally if loosely defined as social work. Each time the government has proceeded thus, however, it has encountered opposition from within the service which it has failed to understand.

It was not until the 1970s that major conflicts arose. These conflicts highlight one of the great problems of modernism – that, as social control theorists have been quick to point out, attempts to control such uncontrollable human activities as crime, sexual behaviour or alcohol and drug consumption are liable to promote more deviance and more repression (see, for example, Young, 1971b; Foucault, 1981: 42; Harris, 1990). Accordingly, though the application of modernist science to social issues is problematic, the contemporary politics of probation has the service trapped within a discourse whereby its future depends on its perceived capacity to prevent people it is supervising from committing crimes. That the service must escape from such demands and engage imaginatively with the uncertainties, paradoxes and surprises it daily encounters is self-evident; equally so are the tactical objections to doing so. Trapped, therefore, between the modern and the postmodern it exudes elements of both, and there is something decidedly postmodern about the ensuing *Angst*.

In England and Wales probation's origins lie in a combination of the common law practices of binding offenders over to be of good behaviour and keep the peace, and granting bail on surety (Grünhut 1948: 299; King, 1958: 1–2; Bochel, 1976: 4–5; McWilliams, 1985; Page, 1992: 6). Under the surety system a willing third party is responsible for producing an offender in court, with financial penalties in the event of failure; but in a process begun by Warwickshire magistrates in the 1820s a prototypical form of probation was conceived by the expedient of extending surety into supervision. People standing surety were asked not only to deliver offenders to court but to supervise and report on them prior to sentence.

Hence, when in 1876 Rainer, a Hertford printer, approached Canon Ellison of the Church of England Temperance Society to suggest extending the society's activities to police courts, the suggestion was not controversial. The system was simple: in suitable cases the court adjourned without passing sentence; the missionary offered supervision for the adjournment period, during which time the offender was normally expected to eschew drink and immorality, and to secure work. The missionary then reported on the offender's attitude and conduct, and if all was well the offender was discharged rather than imprisoned.

From the first the system was a response not primarily to a specific crime but to the offender's general moral behaviour (Harris, 1995). This *extensive* characteristic of probation, this bringing into the public domain aspects of daily life otherwise private – drinking, sexual conduct, family relationships – is crucial to an understanding of probation's tactical utility. It enabled courts to avoid a prison sentence but to fill the vacuum thereby created by instituting a wider-ranging form of tutelage targeted not, as was hard labour, at offenders' bodies but at their daily lives.

Inevitably this tutelage extended into an examination of the conduct of those with whom the offenders came most intimately into contact, involving the injection of morality and order into the private lives of probationers' families. The intervention satisfied everybody, albeit for different reasons: the court was taking constructive action where the correct sentence was unclear but the offender seemed to need help or advice; the probation officer was trusted to get on with an intrinsically rewarding job; and the offender, who might or might not find the intervention helpful, at least avoided prison. But in this pre-modern era, the assumption that these interventions were *effect-ive* depended solely on the word of the officers, who were seldom slow to publicise as moral tracts the fact that they were undertaking God's work – for an early example see Holmes (1900). No independent evaluations took place and there was little doubt in anyone's mind that probation was a good thing and that it 'worked'.

If there is anything anachronistically postmodern about pre-modern probation it is in the paradoxical decisiveness of the equivocation which from the first characterised the system. There was widespread disillusionment with the austere penal theories of the nineteenth century: for many minor and socially deprived offenders prison was a decisive punishment imposed where in-decision was preferable, and probation was a subtle response to the disjunction between decisive penalty and indecisive exigency.

Probation entails shifting responsibility for action from judiciary to executive, relocating the site of intervention from courtroom to office or home, and transferring its justification from the crime to the offender's general conduct. It therefore both offers an alternative to the pains of imprisonment and triggers a return to those pains in the event of infraction. It addresses, in an appropriately ambiguous way, the unfulfilled potential for good of deprived, oppressed or evil people by offering them a gateway to a better life, but initiates sanctions if the gateway be not entered. And it has a story to tell, one epitomised in the epigraph to this section. The epigraph is part of a literary type which, with the Warner Brothers inter-war gangster film in mind, the writer once termed the 'angels with dirty faces' tradition (Harris and Timms, 1993: ch. 3). In the present context, however, it would perhaps be better related to the parable of the prodigal son, with its inclusionary motifs of reformation and forgiveness.

The Probation Service's move from saving souls to the self-conscious professionalism associated with its embrace of psycho-therapeutic techniques has been chronicled elsewhere, albeit with different inflexions (for example, United Nations, 1951, 1954; McWilliams, 1983, 1985), and is not detailed here. Though the shift from a theological to a curative discourse is of significance to the student of probation it had little impact on probation's role in criminal policy and did little to disturb the consensus which characterised that lengthy period when probation functioned, in pre-industrial mode, as an organic village community.

THE 1970s TO THE 1990s: MODERN PROBATION AND BEYOND

Bridlington MP John Townend is backing plans for a tough new approach to young offenders. He welcomed proposals by Home Secretary Michael Howard for a shake-up in the role of the Probation Service. And he hopes it will end the 'scandal' of young tearaways being sent on expensive holidays at the taxpayers' expense. . . . The Minister intends to attract ex-servicemen and retired policemen who will use stricter methods. . . . Delighted Mr Townend hoped the move would end the liberal approach, and lead to more discipline for young offenders. He explained: . . . Young people look up to the leadership and discipline shown by service-men like paratroopers and the SAS. . . . We have had 50 years of the liberal approach, which has done away with the cane, corporal punishment, and the death sentence. Crime figures have gone up and up during that time, and the public are getting fed up of it.

There will be an outcry from do-gooders over the proposed reforms, but they are a minority and I represent the majority.'

(Taylor, 1995)

Phase 1: the 1970s

This prolonged period of *Gemeinschaft* came to an abrupt end in the early 1970s with the attempt of government to introduce rational planning into criminal justice generally and probation specifically. Though it is often claimed that this change was caused by a collapse of confidence in treatment based on the belief that 'nothing works' (Martinson, 1974), this overstates the influence of a research review in an obscure American journal. Martinson's work attracted attention in Britain not because scepticism about the efficacy of interventions in reducing crime was new – see, for example, Powers and Witmer (1951); Meyer *et al.*, (1965) – but because it offered *post hoc* support for ideas moving into prominence for rather different reasons; for a discussion of the politics of Martinson, see Mair (1991).

Nevertheless, in the 1970s the government began to appreciate the central role probation was situated to play in penal policy, and probation expanded as part of the extravagant modernising ambitions of the Heath administration. The years following the Criminal Justice Act 1972 were especially significant. On the basis of recommendations of the Wootton Report (Advisory Council on the Penal System, 1970), the Act introduced five pilot schemes for *community service orders*. These were expeditiously evaluated by the Home Office (Pease *et al.*, 1975; Pease *et al.*, 1977) and expanded: by 1975, 49 out of 56 probation areas had community service schemes and in 1976 no fewer than 8,737 orders were made. Under the same Act four *day training centres* were introduced, with attendance for up to 60 days permitted as a condition of a probation order; *suspended sentence supervision orders* became a new responsibility (by December 1974 nearly 4,000 such orders were in force) (Home Office, 1976: para 8); *hostel places* were scheduled to expand from 58 to 1,650 in a five-year period (see also Haxby, 1978: 245–55); and the service was supervising a massive increase in *parolees*, whose numbers trebled between 1969 and 1971 (Home Office, 1972: para 6).

At the same time probation work involved supervising more serious offenders. After-care cases increased and juvenile supervision declined; social enquiry report-writing shifted significantly from juvenile to adult magistrates' and Crown Courts (Home Office, 1976: Table 2). The pace of workforce expansion increased exponentially up to the mid-1970s when net growth was first restricted (Home Office, 1976: par 14): the six-year period 1970–75 inclusive saw a 50 per cent increase in the probation workforce as well as a reduction in the average caseload of 19 per cent for men and 16 per cent for women (calculated from Home Office, 1976: Appendix F).

Of at least equal significance was the 83 per cent increase in supervisory grades over the same period, involving a fall in the supervisor: main grade officer ratio from almost 5.5:1 to 4.5:1, and a near tripling (from 56 to 158) of deputy and assistant chief officer grades – an indication that the service's traditionally flat and informal supervisory arrangements (there being little concept of management at this time) were giving way to a more hierarchical structure (calculated from Home Office, 1972: Table 2; and Home Office, 1976: Appendix D).

These changes, combined with the growth in the size and cost of the service, made it the object of serious academic and political scrutiny; their cumulative effect was akin to an urbanisation of probation: a small, organic community became complex, organised, impersonal and deviant, its members increasingly estranged both from the courts (McWilliams, 1981) and from one another. As one officer put it in a research interview conducted in 1979:

> Overnight we have accepted a 17.5% salary increase. That's been a great deal about how to buy the probation service off and put us in the law and order league . . . somebody in the Conservative party or the cabinet . . . decided that . . . law and order would include police, the prisons and the probation service . . . somehow politically we're OK. We may not be doing a very good job, somebody needs to say, but [are] part of the fold.
>
> (Fielding, 1984: 163–4)

The broader consequences of these transformations were characteristic of the transition to a *Gesellschaft* community (Tönnies, 1955). Internal dissension increased, and the hitherto staid National Association of Probation Officers found itself unable to cope either with the changes the service was undergoing or the conduct of its own radical members. The Association began to fragment: local ginger groups were formed (some under the umbrella of the NAPO Members' Action Group, founded in 1972); a radical manifesto published by NMAG was repudiated by the Association's leadership in 1977; in the same year NAPO suspended its own London Branch for picketing in the high-profile Grunwick industrial dispute, one considered irrelevant by traditionalists but a site for the expression of working-class solidarity by activists (see Walker and Beaumont, 1981: 93–101). By the mid-1980s the Chairman and General Secretary had been replaced by a Marxist regime led by the co-author of the following passage:

> It is through the union that probation officers can make links with other workers and with wider struggles within the state. Organization in the working-class form of the trade union facilitates these links. It also helps probation officers escape from an esoteric identity as 'the neutral professional' to a recognition of their status as sellers of labour power, having common cause with members of the working-class. These links enable us to connect with, and contribute to, broad and fundamental struggles over social justice, distribution of wealth, eradication of poverty and provision of welfare services.
>
> (Walker and Beaumont, 1981: 194–5)

Probation's most public discourse in the 1970s entailed directly challenging not only the expansion of management grades but also the enhanced accountability to management of main grade staff and the anticipated pressure to impose oppressive modes of control on a working-class clientele with whom radical officers optimistically hoped to express class solidarity. Though such officers comprised only a small minority of probation staff, their objections to the current transformations touched a nerve among non-militant staff, whose agenda was to return to the pre-modern era. These objections crystallised in the mid-1970s around a recommendation that probation's controlling function should be so extended as to include limited powers of detention (Advisory Council on the Penal System, 1974). This was as antithetical to the liberal majority as to the radical minority and a coalition of the two duly saw off the proposal. The radical concern, however, far from seeking to return to an organic past, involved struggling for a liberationist agenda and a horizontal structure of local internal (and only internal) accountability for achieving it:

> In the ideal probation service, the practitioners would have control over their own affairs. Teams would organise the distribution of their work and elected representatives would decide their area

policy. There would still be a need for planners and people to set up projects but this would reflect the expressed need of the practitioners, (*sic*) and representatives would be answerable to their teams.

(NAPO Members' Action Group, 1977; cited in
Walker and Beaumont, 1981: 10–11)

Phase 2: the 1980s and 1990s

By the mid-1980s the political climate could not have been more different. The historical moment when probation officers could feasibly develop a Marxist critique of the state which employed them had passed. Government policy in the public sector now entailed imposing central strategic direction but, supported by slogans such as 'rolling back the state' and 'letting managers manage', decentralising administration to identifiable units and individuals. The performance of these units in meeting policy objectives was monitored by a greatly strengthened evaluative machinery (Henkel, 1991a, 1991b). Incentives such as performance-related pay were introduced; managers were supported by new legal restrictions on trade unions; these in turn paved the way for the introduction of competition in areas where monopoly supply had previously been taken as inevitable. Internal or quasi-markets were introduced, in which provider units competed for contracts in a system of compulsory competitive tendering (LeGrand and Bartlett, 1993). Middle-ranking bureaucrats became managers of budgets to be spent in furtherance of agency mission. In consequence, hitherto heavily unionised public-sector organisations were transformed into internally competitive environments: 'the intention is to turn spenders into managers and to forge a tight relationship between resources and results. Structures are characterized by administrative decentralization, which is seen as a precondition for holding managers to account for what they spend and do' (Gray and Jenkins, 1993: 12).

The 1980s and 1990s saw significant changes for the Probation Service (for a useful discussion, see May, 1991: 37–49). Some commentators take a key (if flimsy) Home Office statement of objectives and priorities as marking a decisive turn in the direction of centralised probation planning (Home Office, 1984; Audit Commission, 1989 *passim* but particularly paragraphs 130–1; National Audit Office, 1989: Part 2). Certainly this paper signalled that the service could no longer operate quasi-autonomously, and that government was intent on creating a coherent criminal justice strategy, with the Probation Service playing a central role in what was then envisaged as a non-prisoncentric policy for property offenders (Harris, 1992).

For the service itself the changes included the surprisingly belated cash limiting of budgets, the introduction of performance-related pay, an obligation to commit 5 per cent of budget to voluntary organisations, the transformation of the probation order into a sentence in its own right, the introduction of National Standards and competences, and the location of training strategy in the Home Office Probation Training Unit. Nevertheless, however seismic these changes may have appeared within the service, they were as nothing compared to those experienced elsewhere. Though there was scope for the creation of a mixed economy within the correctional field, for example, this occurred in very few parts of probation's domain, and the service escaped the introduction of an internal market of the kind on which the National Health Service came to be based. That some structure of this kind did not come about is largely due to the fact that probation was not a policy priority for government during the mid- to late-1980s. At this time government was engaged in the transformations of health, education and the public utilities, and the Home Office in particular was preoccupied with police and prisons. That government is in no position to embark on such a strategy in the mid- to late-1990s seems beyond doubt, though it is a truism to say that predictions have a shorter time span now than at any time in living memory, and that what would have been deemed unthinkable in the 1970s is commonplace in the 1990s – and of course vice versa.

TOWARDS THE FUTURE

Probation makes room for creativity, but it is difficult, and sometimes impossible, to transfer that between posts or individuals.

(Audit Commission, 1991: para 22)

Something in all men profoundly rejoices in seeing a car burn.

(Baudrillard, 1975: 141)

That the probation service has left forever the pre-modern era of informality, reciprocity and agreed purpose characteristic of an organic unit based on mutual affirmation (Tönnies, 1955)[3] is as safe a prediction as one can make in this uncertain world. The modern era of probation has seen an increasing rift with government, the exposure by quantitative measurement of the limitations of its efficiency and effectiveness (Audit Commission, 1989; 1991), ever-increasing political pressure on the service to define itself as government wishes it defined, and a failure on the service's part to agree activities with which it is happy, which it can deliver and which will carry support among the informed public. Accordingly, for much of the 1990s probation has manifested a cowed defensiveness punctuated only by the intermittent but futile protests of a small minority of dissident officers.

A sensible organisational strategy at a time of threat and uncertainty is to keep as many doors open as possible. This predominantly defensive manoeuvre is appropriate to a time when short-term tactics are more important than long-term strategic planning. Certainly it is right for the service to engage enthusiastically with the opportunities which lie before it, aiming to make itself indispensable to courts and other agencies. But at the same time it should ensure that it places its work and the complexities which help define it in the realm of public debate. This entails seizing the initiative and setting an agenda in which it has a realistic chance of success.

Effectiveness is a case in point. There is every reason for the work of probation officers to be scrutinised, and to argue against this is not only untenable but, given government's policies on accountability for public money, whistling in the wind. It is surely proper that what is done should be measured and the outcome of the measurement be disseminated:

> The probation service as a whole still does too little to measure its own effectiveness. And even where they do, they are slow to broadcast and publicise the results . . . it is not enough for a service to do the work, it has to be communicated as well. . . . Far more could be done to 'sell' the service more effectively.
>
> (Audit Commission, 1991: para 21)

For politically and culturally obvious reasons, however, the achievements of probation officers have, since the 1970s, been measured by the yardstick of the modernist scientific discourse. However much researchers protest that matters are more complex than this, the prevailing debate is about 'what works', or how effective probation officers are in changing the criminal behaviour of this or that kind of person by this or that tactic. Probation, which would doubtless be more comfortable as a marginal activity, cannot evade the effectiveness enquiry once it moves centre-stage.

The primacy of this discourse continues notwithstanding the facts that (1) lack of effectiveness has had little bearing on the continued popularity of prison, or on the periodic clamour for the return of capital punishment; (2) as neither probation officer nor offender is an interchangeable variable, and as control groups can do no more than approximate to experimental groups, a personalist social intervention such as probation cannot be replicated like a clinical trial of a pharmaceutical innovation: probation, in other words, cannot be measured independently of the unique way it is conducted and experienced in a given moment; (3) when less than 10 per cent of crimes come to light reconviction rates alone cannot be a meaningful measuring stick; and (4) even should a demonstrable piece of reductionist efficacy be achieved by the Probation Service it would register as scarcely a blip on the criminal statistics as a whole.

None of these caveats, however, implies that probation work cannot or should not be measured. The cost of probation; magistrates' views on its impact on the administration of justice; victim and victim organisations' perceptions of community service and reparative activities; the opinions of the police and members of vulnerable communities on probation's contribution to crime prevention and social support; the comments of offenders themselves on their experience of supervision (albeit that they are strikingly omitted from the contemporary consumerist discourse of the Citizens' Charter) – phenomena such as this can be measured, and there is every reason for the Probation Service to contribute to setting the agenda as to what effectiveness means. (For a brief review of the issues, see Raynor et al., 1994; for an excellent review of the literature on effectiveness see McGuire, 1995).

For example, one useful local study (Raynor, 1988) evaluated a diversionary project in terms of variables which included its impact on local sentencing trends, the tariff location of the probation order, agency workloads and staff attitudes as well as reconvictions; and in a thought-provoking paper a Home Office researcher plots an agenda for measuring effectiveness in relation to such variables as the timing, quantity and nature of reconvictions, diversion from custody, financial costs, sentencer satisfaction, views of offenders and help with problems like accommodation and employment (Mair, 1991).

However, the problem for probation is only in part the management of its present tasks; equally there is the question of the jobs it has lost – those 'softer-end' activities which are hard to measure and, in a socio-political environment based on economic individualism and self-help, harder still to defend. After all, welfare has been withdrawn from more deserving people than offenders, and there could scarcely be a less propitious time than the present to argue that they should be helped other than as part of the service's traditional Faustian pact with government, that probation support will reduce criminal activity.

Hence we return to the point that good work should be publicised and that the narrative dimensions of probation have been submerged in its no-longer-marginal work in the modern world. It will be remembered, however, that narrative and interpretation themselves constitute action, and the nature and consequences of probation officers' narrative interventions have seldom if ever been studied. Story-telling is a ubiquitous part of probation work. Even in offence-focused pre-sentence reports officers explain the otherwise inexplicable, translating confused reality into digestible narrative form (Harris and Timms, 1993: ch. 3); and they chronicle in their agency records the often bewildering, self-destructive, anarchic life-styles of their delinquent charges and their own attempts to deflect them into a more orderly and wholesome *modus vivendi*. Their mission is to render comprehensible experiences and behaviour which would otherwise be – literally – beyond belief.

In short, probation officers are engaged in applying to the inexplicable explanations from their professional repertoire which seem best suited to the case in hand. For many years the sentimentalised image of young offenders as angels with dirty faces helped legitimate a liberal form of neo-classical justice which permitted tolerance where human sympathy spoke louder than the demand for retribution, or where the offender, though within the bounds of legal responsibility, seemed unhinged by psychosocial dislocation.

There is still a place for such formulaic narrative, but its contemporary utility is severely circumscribed. Though there remains a substantial market for formula fiction, as the sales figures of Jeffrey Archer, Barbara Cartland, Jackie Collins and Jilly Cooper show, in the case of offenders the tabloid press has filled any vacuum which might exist with images of very different hue. The portrayal, in a recession which has brought so much hardship and heralded so much crime, of young thugs being taken on luxury holidays by do-gooders understandably provokes angry incomprehension. Though a riposte could be made, it would be unrealistic to believe that this would offset the combination of moral outrage and sound British common sense which the tabloid versions of reality daily reflect.

More generally, however, in a world where social and moral change and technological advance have contributed to a climate where cynicism is *à la mode* and prurience sells newspapers, it would be surprising if the simple moral tale retained its former cachet. The reformed convict telling his story is now metamorphosed into a beneficiary of cheque-book journalism; the priest or youth worker who befriends the deprived young is suspected of paederasty; the social worker's tale of success against the odds with a deprived youngster may unleash enquiries into what the youngster was *really* like, designed to undercut the moral of the story – and as young offenders seldom behave like Dickensian waifs, such undercutting is often not hard to achieve.

For all their need to tell a comprehensible and familiar tale, and for all the contemporary belief that complexity can be boiled down to questions of competence, probation officers do deal with issues of the greatest complexity, as much of the older literature on probation makes plain. It seems important not to forget that, and to do what is possible to publicise it. The case materials available to probation officers are social problems in action, moral mazes which, when articulated by reference to personal experience, do not lend themselves to the flip, unthinkingly punitive solutions to which so much contemporary debate has degenerated:

> Part of social work's dramatic character is that because it is 'real' it does not necessarily follow the formulaic pathways of popular fiction or drama wherein all tensions are resolved, for better or worse, by the final page or curtain. The affirmations of justice, dignity and resilience daily celebrated in popular fiction and mass theatre need not 'come true' in the world of social work: injustices may continue, needs may not be met, interests may be ignored and rights abrogated. Even more characteristically, nothing may be resolved. The comforting predictability of the popular arts, charac- teristically signalled even before we buy the book or enter the theatre by 'signs' ranging from the design of dust wrappers to the tone and content of publicity blurbs is altogether missing in the social worker's world.

(Harris and Timms, 1993: 55)

However politically expedient it may be to do so and however unfashionable to do otherwise, it is not self-evidently progressive or wise to unravel complexity when a *terrible simplification* is likely to result. This is to argue not for obfuscation – there has been too much of that already in probation's history – but for a clear exposition of complex reality. To present this complexity publicly in stories which engage the heart as well as the head may be tactically astute; it may also permit a more recognisable picture of the dilemmas which daily confront courts and the Probation Service to be painted.

The precise nature of these postmodern narratives and the proper sites for and modes of their transmission (which may, in a techno- logically changing era, by no means necessarily be in books or newspapers) must be the subject of further work (though the wheel originally set rolling by Lyotard need not be reinvented: for apposite discussions of postmodern narrative see, among many others, Connor (1989); McHale (1992)). Some likely characteristics can be readily identified, however: they should eschew the 'meta-narratives' of pre-modern moral tales, tales which fit 'reality' into the 'story' and offer tidiness, reassurance, a clear moral and, usually, a happy ending. They should be incomplete, disturbing even, maintaining indeterminacy and, in contemporary mode, interactive, encouraging readers, listeners, viewers or players to create their own texts by defining possible endings, assigning different meanings to the dramas, above all engaging with the problems of action which confront probation officers and sentencers, and which mock the simplistic story-telling which currently enjoys hegemonic status.

The Probation Service deals with far more complexity than is generally appreciated, but the agenda for the public debate today is not drawn up by the service's friends, and the debate itself does not do credit to an advanced European liberal democracy. To change the contours of this debate by changing the literary forms of probation is, in the sense in which this chapter initially defined such matters, to engage in the transformation of probation itself. The alternative is to have that transformation imposed from without.

NOTES

1 The dust wrapper proclaims, 'You owe it to your conscience to read this book'.
2 Here the dust wrapper promises 'The experiences – rich in "human appeal" – of a Juvenile Court and Bow Street Probation Officer'.

3 Lest there be doubt it must be stressed that the use of *Gemeinshaft* and
   Gesellshaft in the context of probation is as an extended metaphor.
   Tönnies uses the terms with a clear sense of historical and geographical
   location.

Chapter 8

The future of social work with older people in a changing world

Judith Phillips

This chapter explores notions of ageing and social work from a postmodern perspective, drawing attention to both changes in social work itself and changing theoretical perspectives in relation to older people. A discussion related to the areas of community care, welfare pluralism and care management is developed with the place of social work in this context being explored. It is argued that for social work to survive and develop within this changing context, it has among other things, to take on more positive images and models of ageing. The concluding section of the chapter reviews ageing in a post-modern framework and the implications for social work with older people.

Dependency and certainty formed the foundations of policy development in modernity in relation to older people. The notion of dependency was articulated in terms of policy through the state provision of care services and via social work through the practice of care-giving to older people. The aim of such policy was to create certainty and hence deliver security to people moving into later life, both through financial provision and care services. The key operators in this process were social services agencies and social workers who almost alone had access to social care provision; their controlling role as gatekeepers to these resources fostered a dependency culture. Conrad (1992) argues that welfare institutions have tended to treat all their older clients as dependent and thus in a negative light: 'This constructed dependency is considered by doctors and social workers as a justification for ever-increased intervention' (p. 80).

In contrast, contemporary developments can be seen potentially to release older people from a negative dependency culture. The assumed tenets on which policies creating a dependency culture are founded have undergone radical change: the family, the world of work and welfare provision are all in a state of flux. Working opportunities over the life course have become less predictable, with secure, lifelong positions becoming increasingly atypical. As employment patterns have changed, so too has retirement with greater flexibility, whether welcomed or not, being provided to many. The formations and structures of 'the family' have been challenged by divorce, single parenthood and reconstituted families. The concept of family is thus in a state of transition due to these alternative models. The promises of security in a cradle-to-grave welfare state have been replaced to a considerable extent by the insecurities of the market place, where those with financial resources have greater access to welfare provision while others are subject to increased isolation and insecurity. This restructuring of the state, however, has also seen the development of more positive approaches to older people, at least for some.

Older people themselves have been in the forefront of recent social policy changes which attempt to promote choice and positive decision-making by empowering consumers. The language of community care, in terms of choice, control, coordination and empowerment, all embodied in recent legislation, seems a positive development. However, the response of social work to these changes has been mixed. Social-work practice has moved from a service-orientated approach to one of assessment of individual need and care management embodying principles of empowerment and choice; however, the interpersonal elements of social work including the important therapeutic relationship have been reduced with, instead, a greater emphasis placed on the management of cases. The future for social work is to respond positively, creatively and in an anti-ageist way to the challenges which are now in evidence.

CHANGES IN SOCIAL-WORK POLICY

The marginalisation of older people in society as a whole has been reflected in both social-work policy and practice over the last two decades, with older people receiving a Cinderella service in terms of the quality of welfare provision and social-work attention (Black *et al.*, 1983). Although the political rhetoric was to keep people at home for as long as possible, there was insufficient financial commitment for this policy and the burden of home-based care was shouldered by informal carers only to be substituted by the state when they could no longer continue. In many instances older people only benefited indirectly from policies focused on other groups.

It is ironic, therefore, that changes to the supplementary benefit rules aimed at youth unemployment in 1979 inadvertently led to a boom in private residential-home placements and increasing state expenditure in private care for older people. Consequent efforts to limit these costs were the driving force towards a more pluralistic form of welfare.

A major change resulting from the National Health Service and Community Care Act 1990 was the heightened profile of 'Community Care' on the welfare agenda. Community care as a label has, perhaps intentionally, lacked clarity: for the mental health lobby it means a move away from large institutions; for financial directors, more cost-effective care; for the bureaucrat, a way of reducing the power of local government (Bamford,1990). To older people community care has been synonymous with increased reliance on the informal sector.

In a social policy context the restructuring of state welfare has had the objective of making as many people as possible self-reliant. The ideal of the provision of welfare and compassionate care-giving has been substituted by that of independence and interdependence in the community. The official aim of the White Paper 'Caring for People' (DoH, 1989) was to enable people to live as normal a life as possible, facilitating the achievement of maximum possible independence, empowering the individual with reference to life-style choices and service utilisation. However, the reality has been different, for choice has been lacking and increasingly support has only been available from family carers (women), which has meant that older people have remained in the community but not under and in conditions of their own choosing.

The independent sector, in contrast to the public sector, has benefited from increased incentives to provide care. In part, the rationale for this has been to stimulate the independent sector to develop community care hence providing wider choice for older people. Local authorities are to act as enablers rather than direct providers, to which end they have been re-organised into purchaser and provider units – a major upheaval in departmental structures, cultures and lines of accountability.

In order to achieve the shift towards the independent sector, a commodification of social relationships is taking place between formal and informal sectors with purchasing and contracting arrangements creating an illusion of securing care provision. Contractual accountability has also resulted in increased monitoring, regulation and inspection; the maintenance of such functions being one of the key features of the 'slimmed-down centre' which has placed greater emphasis on quality management systems (Means and Smith, 1994).

With this increasing fragmentation the need to regulate has increased. The regulation of quality of care and standards of practice has grown with the establishment of inspection units and complaints procedures and with guidelines on residential care provision and practice. Although this can be viewed positively, for many older people it has meant increased uncertainty for both those providing services and those on the receiving end. The introduction of regulation has allowed the state to retreat, selling off its residential care provision, allowing the independent sector to provide services within a framework of registration and inspection. These inspection and registration services, although initially carried out by the state, are increasingly becoming independent themselves.

The establishment of protocols which codify work to be undertaken has been a significant development, notably in the introduction of guidelines concerning the quality of life in residential care and in guidelines regarding the assessment of risk. This again has allowed the state to retreat and set the task for others to undertake.

The concept of risk has dominated the changes in both policy and practice and has been a major distinguishing feature of contemporary developments. The emphasis in social policy, particularly in the last ten years, has increasingly been on the basis of perceived risk. Older people are given services proportionate to their perceived risk, with many local authorities formulating hierarchies or priorities of risk, which require particular responses. Some would argue that risk aversion has taken precedence over flexibility and responsiveness to consumer needs (Bamford, 1990).

Attempts to control uncertainty by administrative definition allows responses and resources to be deployed in a more regular and routine fashion (Howe, 1991). As a consequence, control increasingly rests with management, with practitioner autonomy minimised. Management has hence gained power and significance with the new legislative changes. Langan and Clarke believe that there has been a move to 'transform the character of social services from a welfare agency run by professionals to a customer-centred network of facilities run by managers' (1994: 73)

Howe (1991) argues that by increasing the rules, routines and procedures the manager diminishes the area of professional discretion available to the social worker. Managers, accompanied by information technology, have become the driving force behind current changes.

CHANGES IN SOCIAL-WORK PRACTICE

Social work does not exist independently of its organisational and political contexts. Although the above changes were underpinned by many of the principles embodied in social work and had significant implications for the profession, they were not driven by social workers. The undervalued potential of social work with older people was evident in the lack of attention it received in the legislation, which also reflected the lack of clarity in the aims and roles of social workers in the changing welfare system. Social work means different things to different people – to users and to other professionals it is seen as something they could do themselves. What is expected of social work from all parties, government, users and managers is also often unclear and contradictory. In such circumstances it could be argued that social work with older people has lost sight of its direction.

Social work is, however, about change both at the individual and societal level, and as a profession it has shown great resilience to changes in the past (Stevenson,1994; Preston-Shoot and Agass,1990; Means and Smith, 1994).

> Social workers regularly confront practice dilemmas: the necessity to take difficult decisions, in which there are no right answers, based on a delicate assessment of risk and competing (if not conflicting) rights; and a myriad of pressures, including from within. The result is a complex maze and interaction of personal, professional, interagency and societal dynamics and pressures and potential tangles between service users, social workers, agencies and society.
>
> (Preston-Shoot and Agass,1990: 10)

Social work with older people has always been ambiguous and in this sense there is nothing new in the contemporary challenges. The optimism with which Seebohm was greeted in 1971 did little to clarify the aims and roles of social work with older people. Casework based on psychological theory was seen to have little place in relation to older people; a negative diagnostic and service-orientated approach was followed and much of the work was undertaken by low-paid, unqualified staff, generally women who were described as committing professional suicide by venturing into the field (Phillipson and Walker, 1986). Similarly, dilemmas around the care/control functions of social workers and the rights/risks judgements have been central to professional practice with older people. Presentation of social work through the media has also echoed this ambiguity in role and function, often alienating and confusing older people and their carers (Aldridge, 1994). The changes since 1990 add to these dilemmas, particularly where social workers act as care managers and struggle in the conflict between acquiring value for money and organising effective care packages.

Needs-led assessment and care management are central to the community care reforms. The White Paper and numerous guidance documents refer to the importance of an holistic assessment of need to enhance user choice. In order to achieve this, assessment is to take place in a context of care management, with emphasis on purchasing and coordinating imaginative packages of care rather than directly providing services. Negotiation of the care package with carers and users, together with regular reviews and reassessment, have led to positive approaches. The role of the care manager in overseeing the process of care management, while utilising available resources effectively, is to ensure that older people are restored to their independence in the community with their individual choice promoted. Such an approach implies that services are able to respond flexibly and without duplication. The needs of the user and carer are to be met in such a way that users are empowered in their relationships with assessors and providers.

Despite the enthusiasm with which the changes were greeted, practice tensions and difficulties have arisen. It can be argued that social work has responded negatively to the changes. Separating the assessment from service provision reinforces the view that social work with older people is about providing services – a mechanical operation that can be carried out with the correct forms in a standardised format. The documents place emphasis on functional capabilities and, as Caldock (1993) illustrates, the forms become ends in themselves. The primary emphasis in needs-led assessment is increasingly on assessment documentation (Caldock and Nolan, 1994), with tick boxes and descriptive material taking precedence over analysis of need. Consequently, the focus is on potential negative outcomes and worst-case scenarios.

Hugman also stresses caution when assessing the positive impact of the development of care management. While he argues that care management provides a means for social work with older people to gain a more professional position within the occupation as a whole, because it offers greater autonomy 'coupled with the integration of instrumental and inter-personal skills . . . there is a risk that the instrumental will be stressed over the interpersonal and the management dimension will predominate. Controlling may become the only element rather than being balanced with that of caring' (Hugman, 1994b: 245).

An administrative model rather than a client-centred model could develop. This raises the question of who will be carrying out the work and what it will look like.

New assessment procedures have changed the role of social workers in relation to their clients. Although the terminology (as users, not clients) suggests a positive shift in the locus of power between professionals and older people, the gatekeeping functions of social workers remain. Given the concern, however, over the rising costs of residential care, the panic over numbers of older people in the population and the political context in which social work is developing, it is not surprising that the role of social workers as gatekeepers to resources and as case coordinators takes precedence over their role as caseworkers engaged in a therapeutic relationship. Associated with this is the move towards partnership between worker and user, again welcomed as a positive step. However, this immediately questions the place and validity of the social workers' professional judgement (Cheetham,1993).

The role of others (for example, community psychiatric nurses and occupational therapists) in the traditional professional domains of social work has led to anxiety about function (as well as job security) as each is unclear of who is doing what (Caldock, 1993). Joint work and assessment have shifted the boundaries of other professions overlapping with social work and opening up the social work arena for greater scrutiny and takeover. Care management itself was never intended to be the sole domain of social workers (Audit Commission, 1992: 27), and in fact it can be argued that others more experienced in budget management (a core skill within care management) and contract negotiation should take on the role. Similarly, no longer can social workers hold a claim on counselling as many health-care professionals possess qualifications and skills in this area of practice.

Coordination is required across and between agencies involved in assessing and providing welfare, and joint working and partnerships are seen as vital to the new culture if the 'seamless service' is to emerge. Coordination is a key feature in care management on an individual basis and within the community. Allan (1991) argues that social workers will need not only to network existing communities but should seek to generate new relationships in order to enable families to cope with problems and to set up a base from which reciprocity can flourish.

The very nature of local authority social work is thus being challenged. The contract culture has increased uncertainty – the uncertainty of whether other providers will join the arena of community care and the uncertainty about the range and quality of state provision (Wistow *et al.*, 1994).

Moving to a consumerist culture where social workers are expected to shop around in the private-sector conflicts with the values of many professionals (Phillips, 1992b). A pluralist system of welfare provision is forcing a rethink of current roles and a focus on what constitutes the distinctive contribution of social work's knowledge and skills. According to Means and Smith:

> The biggest challenge faced by central government and local authorities will be to develop community care systems capable of supporting and protecting very vulnerable people in the community with a mixed economy system which requires extensive collaboration between the main statutory agencies of social services, health and housing.
>
> (1994: 230)

The consequence of these processes is a redefinition of social work with older people. Societal norms are changing and social work must adapt to those changes. Some commentators see this as a positive step, with social work in the forefront. Hugman argues that social work and social services have 'a key role to play in shaping the future of professional responses to the needs of older people through their central role in the main changes taking place in the organisation and delivery of community care' (Hugman, 1994b: 238).

How can we understand the sea changes in social work? What is the role for social work with older people? Can social work respond positively and survive, and if so in what form(s)?

ENTER THE POSTMODERN: DECONSTRUCTING THE LIFE COURSE

Discussions related to postmodernity provide a useful framework to consider these developments. If social work is to develop, then it must take on board new, more positive images of ageing, work with diversity and develop a service which does not rest on the concept of dependency.

Some key tenets of postmodernity in relation to discussions of ageing include: deconstruction of the life course; changing images, diversity and pluralisation of life-style; individualism, and the significance of consumption. All of these represent a potentially more positive framework and image of ageing. Featherstone and Hepworth (1989) draw attention to three distinct features of post-modern perspectives on ageing: (1) the cultivation of life-styles and consumerism as people deny the need to slow down; (2) a youthful approach to culture as the media and tourism offer pleasurable stimulations which cut across earlier barriers; and (3) the emergence of new social movements where post-scarcity values are articulated by groups such as women, who act as valid and valued partners in the changing social context.

Understanding changes in a postmodern framework raises the profile of older people, for they are no longer seen as dependent – anything is possible. Care management as a vehicle for social-work practice can act to provide a positive framework for work with older people if the changes in the way older people are constituted are embraced. There should be less concentration on age as a naturally given category and more focus placed on the nature of any difficulties. Hugman argues for 'a focus on the nature of, causes of and solutions to specific difficulties, then a more common response between problems faced in old age and the difficulties faced by younger adults could be developed' (Hugman, 1994a: 123). Deconstructing the life course could lead to more creative and less ageist forms of social work.

Modernity brought about the categorisation and institutionalisation of life stages of childhood, adulthood, middle age and old age. Paralleling these were the 'three boxes of life'- education, work and retirement. The organisation of social work has traditionally been along these lines, with old age associated with decline, disability and the ending of work and education. Postmodern approaches reject these assumptions and argue that there should be 'less emphasis on age specific role transitions and scheduled identity development' (Featherstone and Hepworth, 1989: 144).

Boundaries between these stages are now very fluid. Long-term unemployment, education, redundancy and retirement are seen across the life course, rather than at certain conventional ages. Older people have a greater range of positions and identities, not just as retired and dependent, but as consumers, carers, mature students and in new relationships in work, social, familial and sexual contexts. Both flexibility in life-style and uncertainty are pervasive as people experience the transitions. One example is of older people as consumers entering the market of private residential care where apparent choice is matched by insecurity of tenure and variable standards of quality.

As a result of the deconstruction of age, theories of ageing such as disengagement theory which have been dominant in social work can be rejected as single, overarching explanations of old age. In their place is left a void or confusion of theories and perspectives. Despite this lack of gerontological theory there is one common variable – age. While age is often taken for granted in gerontology there are different ways of expressing this (Bytheway, 1994). Under conditions of postmodernity 'chronological age will continue to be discredited as an indicator of inevitable age norms and life styles with significant new values taking their place' (Bury, 1994: 10).

Such diversity is found within ageing cohorts as well as between cohorts. 'Old age' as a term can no longer be used to describe the experiences of people spanning an age range of 30 to 40 years. 'The pace of cohort differentiation has speeded up, with different age groups reflecting cohort differences in life chances that are created by period specific conditions, policies and economic transformations' (Conrad, 1992: 72).

Similarly, historical continuity also does not exist. 'A post-modernist view of the life course points out that longitudinal studies show little correlation between early- and late-life attributes. Between myself in the past and myself now, there is no continuity, no progress' (Moody, 1993: xxxiii). Time, ageing and the historical past are not entirely real. They represent a social construction that we can change at will, whether in societies or in our individual lives.

Identities are continually shifting and often conflicting as we go through the ageing process – this is not solely as individuals but as cohorts. The postmodernist acknowledges differences in the process of ageing, that it is not a uniform development or experience. There is diversity of subjective experience of ageing and qualitative variations in the life-style of older people. The emphasis is on the *process* of ageing rather than age itself. 'In the context of a postmodernist deconstruction of the life course, the image of the mask of ageing is a further sign of attempts to undermine traditional age related categories' (Featherstone and Hepworth, 1989: 151).

Featherstone and Hepworth assert that the mask of ageing alerts us to the conflict between our outer appearance and functional capacities and the internal subjective experience; to the contrast between the stereotype and the reality; and to the new, more positive language of ageing. This later change is partly a result of the consumer culture, with older people being an important part of the new market.

Society and individuals desire 'successful ageing' with body image, fitness, health and appearance ascribed great importance. Reassessment and commodification of the body are key features of postmodernism, with the notion that the inevitability of decline can be controlled. Shilling suggests that 'bodies become malleable entities which can be shaped and honed by the vigilance and hard work of their owners' (1993: 5).

In relation to behaviour and experience, potentially 'anything goes'. This can also be true of health and welfare situations as it is for life-style as Gubrium's analysis of Alzheimer's disease illustrates. The incommunicable – experiences that some say cannot be put into words – are conveyed according to culturally recognisable codes (Gubrium,1988). The changed vision of old age, as reflected in the film *Cocoon*, 'gives way to a postmodern ethos of playful possibilities and denial of limits' (Moody, 1993: xxxiii).

This positive imagery of old age stands in contrast to the modern view of old age as a time of decline and neglect, problem-orientated and age-conscious. No longer can there be a standard image of old age. The grandmother stereotype portrayed in Victorian art and literature is just one way of experiencing age. Phillipson (1994) argues that new alternative forms of ageing are driven by reflexive, risk-taking forms of identity. As a result there are new social identities in to be constructed.

There are two ways in which social work can respond to these cultural changes. In assessment, the strengths and resources of the person should be considered in addition to their needs and any specific risks. Positive aspects of ageing must be reinforced rather than models of decline. This requires change within social work, for many of the new tools of assessment rely on tick boxes and are 'dominated by a pathology or difficulty perspective with little opportunity to highlight users and carers existing strengths, potentials and desires' (Caldock and Nolan, 1994: 2).

Second, determining the level of risk in practice will, however, be an increasing feature. With growing numbers of older people living longer there will be a concentration on a high-priority group – namely concentration on Laslett's fourth age – a phase of final dependence, decrepitude and death. Consolidation of skills and expertise in decision-making regarding residential care and issues of vulnerability will be important. This will be increasingly significant where frail older people have no relatives to act on their behalf. The focus will be on developing assessment and designing creative and flexible packages of care for a select group of high-risk older people. Other groups will have little or no eligibility or access to a service. Within this context it is vital that a critical awareness of the difficulties faced by older people with health and social needs develops alongside an emphasis on the positive aspects of ageing.

This will require, for example, the development of social models of ageing in multi-disciplinary assessments rather than employing a medical model. 'Clearly, to meet this requirement the emphasis on services would have to be on the enhancement of ordinary life rather than on perceptions of deficit' (Hugman, 1994a: 123).

It is crucial to promote positive images of ageing even when welfare services are involved – positive choices need to be highlighted in relation to the type and quality of care required; forms of empowerment developed among Alzheimer sufferers are one example. Counselling focusing on change rather than maintenance should form a basis of working with older people. If the definition of risk is to incorporate a user perspective in its determination and how it might be minimised, then more positive approaches are required. The skill for the social worker is 'in moving the focus beyond what may be their limited horizon requiring a sensitive, exploratory approach which validates the carer and user perspective but integrates with it the knowledge and skills of the practitioner' (Hughes, 1993: 361).

DIVERSITY AND LIFE-STYLE

Diversity of life-style will also challenge ways of working with older people. New forms of relationships within and without the family will have consequences for later life, not specifically in care-giving and receiving but for experience in general, as divorced, reconstituted families, and fictive kin along with other forms of partnerships enter the framework. Postmodernism heralds the plurality of cultures and life-styles previously marginalised and excluded from the debate – lesbian elders and black perspectives among others.

The redefinition of family has significant implications for older people in terms of negotiating care responsibilities for 'the role of the family in the care of the dependent is complicated, varied and ambiguous' (Baldock, 1994: 187).

The regrouping of families has led to a multiplicity of step-grandchildren in fragmented and complex family trees. Accompanying this is a plurality of living arrangements, where shared care of children and dependent adults between different households at different times is one way of negotiating differentiated life-styles.

The fragmentation of families through separation, divorce, geographical distance and mobility has been experienced on a large scale by older people today. Certainties about care-giving are no longer available as kinship obligation has to compete with other pressures and employment. As women increasingly enter the workforce and attempt to balance work and care-giving, their ability to manage both roles can be put under considerable strain. At the same time, men increasingly share time in terms of paid employment and activities in the home. Assumptions and experiences within the family are different as a consequence. A greater range of identities is also experienced within the family relationship as carers enter the labour market (unexpected combination) and fictive kin take the place of sons and daughters (hyperreal). The reconstitution of the 'family' also reflects shifts to other networks based on gender, race and ethnicity rather than on age.

Over the last decade family and older people have been discussed in the social-work literature purely as dependent within a care-giving relationship. Social workers will need to broaden their perspective to encompass the diversity of family life, viewing carers with needs of their own rather than purely as resources (Twigg and Atkin, 1994). The potentials and strengths of older people as carers and workers also need to be highlighted rather than a negative focus be given to their difficulties and problems. Although care management has gone some way in recognising this, social work has yet to develop more creative strategies and partnerships – for example, with employers in designing strategies for helping working carers and with private-sector providers in securing genuinely flexible services.

Postmodern analyses point to a shift away from traditional dependency relationships between professionals and clients towards models of common ownership in assessment of need and packages of care (Caldock and Nolan, 1994). The failure of professional expertise and knowledge to ameliorate problems has created uncertainty in social work and has led to the promotion of partnerships between professionals and users and carers. Although this is seen as a way of empowering users, there is still uncertainty about the location of power as social workers still act as the gatekeepers to resources. Many older people also have few ideas of their rights and only a limited understanding of assessment (Caldock and Nolan, 1994). A challenge for social work is therefore to engage in meaningful partnerships with older people based on their skills of advocacy and negotiation in a relationship of trust.

A major area of social change is in relation to consumption and the increased emphasis on individualism. The emphasis on individualism reflects in part changing values in terms of family and self. There is less time involved with the extended family and more on consumption. This redefinition of the position of the individual can be seen as a long-term process, which in turn has redefined the family. As a result of this, some would argue there has been an aversion to long-term commitment, not only in relation to bonds of marriage but to older people within the family (Conrad, 1992). There is also a tension between commitment and maximisation of self-interest, particularly as more women move into the labour market.

It is incorrect, however, simply to assume that an increased emphasis on individualism necessarily undermines the family and the community. The situation is much more complex. Older people value the commitment of the family and reward long-term support by the family in relation to inheritance (Finch and Wallis, 1994). Similarly, 'the individualism of making something of oneself and putting the family first can produce a stable order of partnership and support during retirement' (Jordan, *et al.*, 1994: 224).

Clearly, however, the dissolution of common value orientations, as Conrad (1992) describes, is of significance. Family and communal meaning and security are lost – secular and individualistic values, the self and body become more important than shared values. The loss of common social meanings for life and death may be felt more acutely by older people. Although death is certain, the lack of certainty in a life thereafter poses insecurity for many older people.

Older people in general are seen in the market place. Their styles of consumption play a significant role in defining their identities, both socially and personally. Patterns of consumption, however, are increasingly segregating groups of older people. Wealthy older people – whoopies – have designer life-styles and a certain niche in the market. For example, the growth of private sheltered housing, insurance schemes for the over fifties and Saga holidays cater for different life-styles for a select group.

One of the advantages of such consumerism is that older people are seen in a valued role after retirement and share a common experience across generations. Featherstone and Hepworth (1989) argue that the fifty plus age marketeers are playing an influential role in the social reconstruction of models of positive ageing. The majority of older people, however, have not benefited in the consumer boom. Consumerism is a limited group experience, reserved for those with financial resources and the opportunities to participate in the market. This group does not generally feature to any considerable extent among social work's clientele. Within the reorganised social services, however, the needs of older people are being commodified to be 'dealt with on the basis of market forces' (Hugman, 1994a: 122). Those without resources are therefore further penalised and marginalised.

CONCLUSIONS

If social work is to survive, it needs to challenge the negative notion of ageing described above and be an advocate for those who are marginalised in the market place. Social workers will also need to come to terms with the diversity of need and provision of welfare, and develop appropriate and flexible responses involving negotiation with the independent sector. The task facing social workers in the 1990s is to develop an appropriate role for themselves in the welfare market while grounding their practice firmly in social-work values. Concurrent to this, social workers must develop a system of accountability which does not lose sight of the needs of the clients and their support systems (Phillips, 1992). If social work is to survive, then it needs to grasp this challenge. Uncertainty is inherent in social work and the context in which it operates; doubts abound about the scope and scale of welfare pluralism (Bamford, 1990) and the extent to which social work is practised within it. The role of social workers as counsellors will need to be reintroduced and highlighted if all needs are to be met.

Later life does bring limits, both physiological and social, and this poses ethical dilemmas. One of the central tensions is that, while there are various movements contributing to a more positive image for older people, age brings with it risks of dependency. Those risks are increasing with a growing number of older people. Governmental, administrative, managerial and public attention has increasingly been given to the finite nature of all resources. The debate has focused around the issues of generational conflict and competition between young and old over such resources. Images of conflict raises uncertainty over the long-term care needs of older people. Positive views of ageing may, ironically, detract from the availability of resources. Welfare professionals also have a vested interest in perpetuating the dependency culture and the modernist view of old age as one of neglect in order to justify their intervention and to direct resources to older people. Ageing therefore is not just a function of the ability to mobilise resources (Bury, 1994). As people experience transitions in the life course they may be hindered by the lack of power or the dominance of one group or another. For example, power structures in the process of admission to and within residential care can often disempower older women; the influence of relatives and social workers in the decision-making process has significant implications on when, where and how older people move to residential care over which they may have little choice, control or independence (Phillips, 1992).

Areas of uncertainty exist within social work in relation to what role it should play in the postmodern world. However, it will be in areas where difficult ethical and legal decisions are to be made that social work will continue to have a key role. Areas where people need protection against risk, where complex decisions need to be made which rely on professional judgement and not on standardised proformas and situations where there is conflict between different parties will require interventions by social work. Social workers will have a key role to play in resolving such conflicts, sometimes via the use of statutory interventions.

New agendas are emerging in social work as a consequence of these changes. Traditionally, work with older people hinged around loss and bereavement, together with experiences of admission to residential care. As social work moves into uncertainty it needs to embrace realistic but positive approaches to working with older people. The importance of body image, for example, may be an essential part of work with older people, who may require counselling. Exploring the nature of risk will also be an important area of work for social workers. Postmodern perspectives are useful in exploring the changes which are taking place in social work with older people. If social work is to survive it has to be flexible and respond to these changes with more positive images of older people and with positive strategies for empowering in a mixed economy of welfare.

Chapter 9

Social work with children and families

From child welfare to child protection

Olive Otway

The abuse of children has been subjected to lengthy public, political and professional debate, particularly since its 'rediscovery' as a social problem in the early 1970s (Parton, 1985). Professionals are continually involved in intense debates concerning the manifestation of child abuse, its cause and extent and how the multi-agencies involved should and can respond. At the core of the debate are those agencies such as health and welfare and the legal profession which have a mandate and responsibility to react. The main focus of this chapter is to explore the important changes in the relationships of the central players involved in the arena of decision-making and analyse how this is affecting social-work practice with children and families.

In the 1960s, child abuse was viewed as essentially a medico-social problem; today, it is usually seen as a socio-legal problem, where legal specialisation takes charge. In the past, the professionals were concerned with diagnosing, curing and preventing the 'disease' or syndrome. Today, the emphasis is placed on investigating, assessing and examining the 'evidence'. This chapter explores the decisive factors that have influenced and revolutionised the policies and practices we now label 'child protection' and how these have led to an increasingly bureaucratised and regulated way of working with families. The practice that this results in may increasingly be marginalising front-line practitioners from their clients and from their own skills and ethical base.

The Children Act 1989 and the Criminal Justice Act 1991 together with the guides, *Working Together under the Children Act 1989* (DOH, 1991a) and the *Memorandum of Good Practice on Video Recording with Child Witnesses for Criminal Proceedings*, (Home Office, 1992), were produced following a succession of contradictory arguments concerning how professionals should respond to the dilemma of child abuse. What the legislation and the guides confront is a problem which has been a predominant worry for the liberal state since the mid-nineteenth century. The problem is this: how can we formulate a legal basis for the authority to intervene in family life in order to protect children, but which prevents all families from becoming clients of the state, while at the same time presenting this legislation as applicable to all (Parton, 1991)?

There was clearly a need following the child abuse enquiries of the 1970s and 1980s for a new set of practices and priorities among social-work professionals. However, while the legislation and subsequent guidelines are viewed by some as a solution to the problem of child abuse, others believe that it has contributed to the bureaucratisation of the organisations and the response of social-work professionals (Howe, 1992), and in the technicalisation of the role of social work.

The gender bias inherent in the framing of the social-work agenda throughout the 1970s and 1980s, and specifically within the context of abuse enquiries, has added to this bureaucratisation (Hudson, 1992). This bias is also inherent in the framing and execution of the new guidelines and policies and has come about by a masculinisation of the managerial role and hierarchy within Social Service Departments. As in the area of child sexual abuse, where men quickly dominated both the discourse and positions of power within the emerging 'industry', likewise in the field of child protection, where women's experiences and values are being replaced by those of men and business.

Finally, it will be argued that these movements are detrimental to the profession and, most importantly, for its service-users on grounds of both efficiency and quality.

THE GROWTH OF CHILD ABUSE AS A MEDICO/SOCIAL PROBLEM WITHIN THE FRAMEWORK OF 'WELFARISM'

Following the Second World War, the creation of the child care service in England and Wales can be seen as an example of the increase and rationalisation of social interventions affiliated to the establishment of 'welfarism' (Rose and Miller, 1992). A central tenet of welfarism concerned the endeavour to join the fiscal calculative and bureaucratic capacities of the state in order to motivate national growth and well-being via the encouragement of social responsibility and the mutuality of social risk and was premised on notions of social solidarity (Donzelot, 1988).

The evolution of social work with children and families, initially under the patronage of the Children's Departments following the Children Act 1948, in the context of welfarism, was infused with optimism, for it was believed that demonstrable improvements could be made in the lives of individuals and families following discerning professional involvement. Social work reflected a supportive social mandate, which deemed that a beneficial and sympathetic involvement with the family was required, so enabling the state and the family to work in partnership to ensure that children experienced the suitable conditions needed in which to develop.

This optimistic growth and institutionalisation of social work in the context of welfarism resulted in the establishment of Social Services Departments following the Local Authority Social Services Act 1970. The Act mirrored the philosophy of the Seebohm Report (1968) which assumed that social problems could be surmounted through state intervention by professional experts who possessed social scientific knowledge and skills in relationships, and visualised a liberal, widespread service available to everyone and with wide community support.

The agreed view which underpinned the development of social work with children and their families during this time had a number of levels. There was a belief that the interests of the social workers and, therefore, the state were similar to those who became clients. When a family received intervention from a social worker this would be via casework, help and guidance, and if a young person did come into state care this was believed to be in their best interests. The law, at this time, was not considered to be significantly relevant to social work, as it did not aid the development of skills and techniques when working with families. The courts and the legal system appeared to have a secondary role for providing the mandate needed in therapeutic interventions. The police were also viewed as marginal and a potential source of difficulty (Baher et al., 1976).

The conceptualisation of child abuse and the explanation of it following its modern 're-discovery' was governed by the 'disease' or public health model (Parton, 1985; London Borough of Brent, 1985: 88). There was an assumption that child abuse was an illness and that clinical medico/scientific approaches were the best way of identifying, explaining and responding. Medical professionals, with social workers, were seen as being able to provide the necessary skills to prevent and cure child abuse. In medical parlance child abuse was given its own diagnostic category. The cause of the disease was seen to be the parents and its symptoms were exhibited in their relationship with the child.

The central role of research, at this time, was to discover the traits that distinguished the 'abusing family' from the 'non-abusing family', and the practitioner was expected to be aware of these 'known characteristics of child abuse' and to be able to identify them and act accordingly (London Borough of Brent, 1985: 100). This method affected the formation of official policy and practice during the 1970s and early 1980s. The process of child-abuse management was effectively set up with the emergence of a Department of Health and Social Security circular (DHSS, 1974) in April 1974 following the Maria Colwell enquiry. It stressed the requirement for teamwork and 'strongly recommended' the creation of case conferences, area review committees and registers. The involvement of paediatricians, general practitioners, health visitors and social workers was considered crucial and the Social Services Department, as the statutory child-care agency, was focal. The police at this stage were not seen as vital. It was a further circular in 1976 (DHSS, 1976) which recommended that a senior police officer should be included on all area review committees and case conferences. Although there is an indication of a tension and different approaches between health, welfare, law and order agencies, the medico/scientific model held the commanding role.

THE VOICES OF DISSATISFACTION

The optimism apparent in social work, and the welfarist child-care system more generally, received several critiques from the mid-1970s, increasing in depth during the 1980s. Apprehension emanated from within social work itself and involved the apparent poor quality of child-care practice in the recently established Social Services Departments. The poor quality of skills and the inability to exploit the emphasis on prevention in the 1960s were the dominant concerns of the National Children's Bureau Working Party (Parker, 1980). Such concerns were similarly shared in the various DHSS and Economic and Social Research Council research studies (DHSS, 1985b) and the Parliamentary Select Committee (Social Services Committee, 1984).

The effect of such criticisms undermined the optimistic welfare consensus in child care. The growth of the women's movement from the 1960s onwards and the consequent recognition of violence in the family resulted in the acknowledgement that not only may the family not be a haven for all its members, but that its less powerful members – namely, women and children – were suffering a range of abuses from the male members. A lot of the early critical analysis emanated particularly from feminist practitioners, and was aimed primarily at improving the position of women. It was only in the 1970s, with the increasing awareness and knowledge of sexual abuse, that attention was directed to the circumstances of the children (C. Parton, 1990; N. Parton, 1990). Such critiques brought about a rudimentary questioning of the family 'blood-tie' and the growth of the children's rights movement (Franklin, 1986; Freeman, 1987–88).

Towards the end of the 1960s, there emerged a civil liberties critique which focused upon the nature of the intervention in people's lives that was permitted to take place unchecked, in the name of welfare (Taylor *et al.*, 1980; Unsworth, 1987). Initially, such views were associated with critiques specifically related to parental rights' resolutions (Morris *et al.*, 1980; Geach and Szwed, 1983).

It was during the mid-1980s that the parents' lobby achieved its most coherent voice, with the creation of Parents Against Injustice (PAIN). While its direct influence and lobbying upon the Children Act may be considered minimal, it did assist in drawing up and vocalising some of the chief concerns raised during the events in Cleveland and subsequently in Rochdale and Orkney (even though it is not clear whether the parent lobby effectively represented the voices of non-abusing parents in what were predominantly issues concerning sexual abuse, as the issue of gender has never been allowed a public airing in official inquiries). Consequently, the rights of parents and of children to remain at home, undisturbed by state intervention, were placed on the political and professional agendas. As a result state intervention, through the practices of health and welfare professionals, as well as parental violence, was recognised as being actively and potentially abusive.

CHILD-ABUSE INQUIRIES

Major criticisms of policy and practice in child care and the competencies of social workers was called into question in the child-abuse inquiries that followed the deaths of several children. It was the death of Maria Colwell that produced the first in a long line of inquiries (Secretary of State, 1974; Parton, 1985). However, such inquiries gained a new level of intensity during the mid-1980s via the inquiries into the deaths of Jasmine Beckford (London Borough of Brent, 1985), Tyra Henry (London Borough of Lambeth, 1987) and Kimberley Carlile (London Borough of Greenwich, 1987). It was public enquiries which provided the forum for political and professional debate concerning the response to child abuse. These inquiries took place in a very public way and received full media attention (Franklin and Parton, 1991; Reder, *et al.*, 1993). The inquiries provided detailed descriptions of what had gone wrong in the individual situations but also remarked critically on the current state of policy and practice more generally and made recommendations as to what could and should be accomplished (DHSS, 1982; DOH, 1991b).

Up until the mid-1980s the thirty-five inquiries had all been concerned with the deaths of children at the hands of their parents or caretakers. Many of the children had been in the care of the local authority but 'returned home on trial' or were under the legal supervision of social workers. All the children died as a result of physical abuse and neglect and often suffered emotional neglect and failure to thrive. The child-care professionals, particularly social workers, were seen to have failed to protect the children, with fatal repercussions.

Rather than view the deaths as occurring solely from the individual incompetencies of the professionals involved, the incompetencies were generally perceived as particular examples of the current state of policy, practice, knowledge and skills and the way systems performed and inter-related. The need to reformulate the management of the problem at the inter-agency, agency and individual case level was conceded (Pound, 1991).

The inquiries pointed to failures in inter-agency and inter-professional cooperation and coordination (Hallett and Birchall, 1992). Significantly, however, social workers were seen as too gullible and trusting of parents, therefore failing to focus on the well-being of the child and failing also in using the statutory authority entrusted to them.

The events in Cleveland and the ensuing report (Secretary of State, 1988) supplied a separate collection of concerns and circumstances and apparently provided a different set of opinions of what was wrong and how professionals should react. It seemed that professionals, paediatricians as well as social workers had failed to accept the rights of parents and intervened impetuously and in an unwieldy way where there were concerns about sexual abuse in family life. Although the cause of the crisis may be essentially placed in inter-agency and inter-professional misunderstandings, resulting in poor cooperation and communication, the legal framework and social-work practice in child-abuse work were again prioritised. It was acknowledged that the law itself needed to be altered, but also that it had to be recognised that professionals should be much more cautious and answerable when collating the 'evidence', legally framed, for what comprised sexual abuse and child abuse more generally. It was not simply a question of obtaining the correct balance between family autonomy and state intervention but also getting the correct balance between the power, discretion and responsibilities of the judicial, social and medical experts and agencies. Here the judicial and the legal aspects were central and therefore the main focus should be investigation, identification and consideration of forensic evidence. It was seen as critical that the law and legal thinking be involved in the decision-making which had such fundamental consequences for children and parents, and hence the family, which was viewed as being essentially undermined by the professionals involved in the investigations in Cleveland.

Curiously, the central question of gender and more specifically the social construction of male authority and its abuse within families was never seriously questioned by the Cleveland Report. Whereas the net result of the inquiries into the physical violence of men towards children within families was to seek to invest more powers (albeit bureaucratic ones) in the social worker's right to intervene in family life, the Cleveland Report, in denying the centrality of abusive male power in the crisis, chose to confirm the state's view of the authority of fathers in families as more important than that of protecting children.

Men and women who were parents or carers of the children involved were viewed as sharing common and equal agendas – namely, to protect their children from a bullying and interfering, female social-work and medical profession.

One of the later consequences of this fundamental omission has been the lost opportunity of empowering non-abusing parents (generally women) through policies and procedures that place them at the forefront of child protection intervention. It has been left to individual local authorities to devise their own practice guidelines (Otway and Peake, 1994).

An overwhelming criticism built up of the processes that had sought to transform these families from their 'dysfunctional' mode to a 'healthy' one. Instead of attempting to work therapeutically with families, the focus of social-work intervention should be to protect children from violence, and because the language used to define these new roles was more akin to that used by the Police force than a caring profession, words like 'investigation', 'assessment', 'dangerousness', 'evaluation', 'forensic evidence' and so on became commonplace.

Howe summarises the changes:

> Social workers would have to become investigators and not family caseworkers. Managers would have to become designers of sur-veillance systems and not casework consultants. Parents would have to become objects of inquiry whose behaviour could be predicted and not people whose skills could be improved. The shift is from therapy and welfare to surveillance and control.
>
> (1992: 497)

It was lawyers who were subsequently seen as crucial to decision-making, with social-work practice being watched and evaluated through legal scrutiny. The law, developing in importance, was not only interested in social workers' and others' actual awareness of the statutes but also strove to change attitudes and the course of practice in order to protect children. In effect, the need to collect evidence in a prescribed way has meant that the discretion of social workers has been hugely curtailed. Parts of the Children Act 1989 – for example, Section 47 – have further stressed that the need to protect children outweighs the more preventive messages given by the Act.

Efforts to justify and improve the multi-disciplinary frameworks, the expanding importance placed on the legal conditions of the work and on enhancement of practitioners' knowledge of the signs and symptoms suggestive of child abuse were at the hub of the recom-mendations to improve the protection of children. As a result, while quite different in their social location and their focus of concern, there was a growing set of constituencies developing from the late 1970s which criticised the post-war welfarist consensus in relation to child care and the medico/scientific dominance in relation to child abuse. These were most forcefully pronounced in and via child-abuse inquiries. Arguments appeared for a greater reliance on individual rights firmly located in a reformed statutory framework where there was an increased emphasis on legalism. Within this emphasis, the rule of law, as ultimately judged by the court, takes priority over those considerations which may be viewed by the professional 'experts' as optimally therapeutic or 'in the best interests of the child'.

However, these Reports are as important for what they did not cover as to what they recommended. The way that the problems are framed and the methods of investigation used were invariably bureaucratic. They reflected the rational and systematic views of the government departments that determined what was to be included in their brief. The view that anything is manageable as long as it can be understood and categorised led to recommendations that themselves stressed more efficient use of administrative and technological solutions.

In many respects, therefore, the results of the official inquiries reflected both the nature of the enquiries themselves and to a large extent the maleness of their terms of reference and methods. As such, the Cleveland Report was viewed as a crisis of management, not as a crisis for children, and the recommendations reflected this view. If the inquiry had considered the issue of gender, it might have been that the need for therapeutic as opposed to legalistic intervention in the lives of families could have been placed on the social-work agenda.

RECENT LEGISLATIVE CHANGES AND PRACTICE GUIDELINES

The central principles of the Children Act 1989 sought an approach to child care based on negotiation with families and involving parents and children in agreed plans (Newton and Marsh, 1993). The guidance and regulations encourage professionals to work in partnership with parents and young people. Similarly, the Act strongly encourages the importance of supporting families, with children in need, in preventive work, thereby keeping care proceedings and emergency interventions to a minimum. It is apparent that professionals involved with families need to be honest and open and that working agreements are central in making clear the roles and responsibilities of those involved (Owen and Pritchard, 1993).

An objective of the Act was concerned with attempting to make both the content and operation of the law seem equitable for all. The Act was attempting to construct a new consensus, or what was often referred to as a new set of balances, related to the respective roles of various state agents and professionals and the family in the upbringing of children. Consensus is central to the Act. While it may be inappropriate to see the Children Act as a direct consequence of Cleveland and other child-abuse inquiries, it was consideration about how to respond to child abuse that was at its core.

Concerns about child protection were dominant, and the emergence of individual rights and legalism framed what constituted the 'welfare of the child'. Another important component to emerge was the criteria to be used for making decisions. The assessment of 'high risk' dominated (Parton and Parton, 1989a). In the Children Act 'high risk' is formulated in terms of 'significant harm'; for the criteria for state intervention for care proceedings, supervision orders and emergency protection orders is 'that the child concerned is suffering, or is likely to suffer significant harm' (31(2) (a)). For the first time the criteria for state intervention includes a prediction of what may or is likely to occur in the future.

Since the mid-1970s the concept of dangerousness or the classification of 'high risk' has become a primary theme in discussions of reforming systems of state social regulation more generally (Bottoms, 1977). Assessments of actual or potential 'high risk' become the central concern and activity. However, in a context where the knowledge and research for assessing and identifying 'high risk' is itself disputed and where the consequences of getting that decision wrong are monumental, it is not seen as suitable to leave that decision to the health and welfare experts alone. The decisions and the accountability for making them need ultimately to be lodged within a legal framework and to be based on forensic 'evidence'. Thus, while assessments of high risk are pivotal they are framed in terms of making judgements about what forms actual or likely 'significant harm'. The implication is that the legal oversight and the identification and weighing of evidence cast a shadow throughout child-abuse work and child care more generally. However, it is conditional on a range of safeguards set in place via the need to work in partnership with children and families and 'working together' with a range of agencies and professionals.

Law and order agencies are now involved in a way that was not evident previously. This is apparent in relation to the central role now played by the police and the legal profession as outlined in the guide *Working Together under the Children Act 1989* (Home Office, 1991).

The central investigating statutory agencies are now the police and

Social Services, and it is seen as imperative that there is an early 'strategy discussion to plan the investigation, the role of each agency and the extent of joint investigation' (para 28). It is stated that such cases 'involve both child care and law enforcement issues' (para 5.14.4). Central to the process is the completion of a social assessment, drawing on the Department of Health publication (1988) *Protecting Children: a Guide for Social Workers Undertaking a Comprehensive Assessment.* It became clear during the 1980s that it was not enough to justify and formalise the mechanisms for inter-agency working and the framework of the law alone. If 'risk' was going to be identified and weighed, it was necessary to improve and clarify the role of the social assessment – for which social workers were significantly responsible. David Pithers has pointed out, 'the guide addresses the key issue of whether a family is considered safe for a child, or whether it can be made safe, or whether it is so potentially dangerous that alternatives have to be found' (Pithers, 1989: 18).

Protecting Children strove to ensure that the rationalisation of inter-agency procedures was matched by attempts to develop practice skills in the assessment of individual cases. It accepted that child protection work could never be risk-free and that there were no easy formulas for success in terms of outcome. It outlined the processes that should be followed and the questions that should be asked in carrying out an assessment which was systematic in order to provide an improved foundation for decision-making. It would also 'provide opportunities for more effective supervision and management of the social work task' (DoH, 1988: 3).

The guide established the process of assessing 'high risk' which is central to child protection work. The large number of questions listed do not in themselves provide a formula for identifying high risk but rather provide a basis for making professional judgements about viability in the context of what is known, the potential for change and the resources available to assist such change. The social worker is to make recommendations on the basis of 'the professional judgements about the relative weightings of the various considerations of factors' (DoH, 1988: 69).

The guides develop and formalise the contemporary nature of child protection work. Social workers are operating not as counsellors or therapists but as case managers, coordinating and taking central responsibility for assessing 'risk' and monitoring and assessing change. This takes place in a context where procedures set out the mechanism for carrying out the work and thereby, potentially, making policy and practice clear and accountable where this accountability is essentially to the parents and, to a lesser extent the children, on the one hand, and the court, on the other. This is not to assume that all cases go to court, but that the court and legal scrutiny increasingly frames child protection work and what constitutes child abuse.

These developments were further reinforced with the new practices and procedures established following the Criminal Justice Act 1991 and the *Memorandum of Good Practice* (Home Office, 1992). More than ever the mechanisms for gathering evidence in relation to both the processes of prosecution of offenders and the protection of the child have been combined.

The *Memorandum of Good Practice* attempts to bring together 'the interests of justice and the interests of the child' (1992, foreword). It was widely acknowledged that the criminal courts were not conducive to hearing the evidence of children who were usually the key witness in prosecution cases. Not only were children not believed, but the procedures for giving evidence, examination and cross-examination could be experienced as abusive to children (Mellor and Dent, 1994). In 1988 the government decided to allow child witnesses to give evidence from outside the courtroom via a special television link and to ease the rules about child witnesses. This was extended in the Criminal Justice Act 1991. For the first time video recordings of earlier interviews with police and social workers could be played to the court as part of the trial. The *Memorandum of Good Practice* attempts to provide guidance about how this may be attempted which, while sensitive to the child, ensures that the evidence so produced will stand up in a criminal court.

The nature of evidence and the standard of proof under civil proceedings established by the Children Act 1989 is different from and less than that constituted in criminal proceedings under the Criminal Justice Act 1991. It appears that the two may be becoming confused and that it is the latter which is pre-eminent and structures the former (Wattam, 1992). The move towards merging the role of the police and social workers in investigations has had the effect of raising the threshold for identifying what comprises a child protection case. In many respects, therefore, the legalism already set in place by the Children Act 1989 is further emphasised. For some this concentration on legalism with respect to children as witnesses in criminal proceedings is leading to further distress to young victims of sexual assault and therefore decreasing the likelihood of criminal convictions for those who are the perpetrators (Flin and Tarrant, 1989).

CHILD PROTECTION WORK IN THE 1990s

The emphasis on the need to identify 'high risk' in a situation where notions of working together are set out in increasingly complicated yet specific procedural guidelines and where the work is framed by a narrow emphasis on legalism and the need for forensic evidence helps us understand the contemporary nature and significance of child protection work. Work in this area from the mid-1980s onwards has increasingly been re-framed in the language of child protection. There are now child protection strategy meetings, child protection case conferences, area child protection committees and child protection registers. Likewise, many Social Services Departments have child protection officers and teams, while Health Authorities and Trusts and police forces have staff specifically designated as specialising in child protection. The growth of training in various aspects of child protection has also increased.

Several influences have reinforced this. First, the definition of child abuse has been officially broadened to include neglect, physical abuse, sexual abuse, emotional abuse and, recently, organised abuse (Dingwall, 1989: DoH, 1991a).

Second, public, professional and political awareness has grown considerably. This is revealed in the numbers of referrals to Social Service Departments, the number of children's names placed on child protection registers and the high numbers of those who call help lines. The year 1988 saw the first collection of national statistics which summarised trends in the registration of cases on registers. A major conclusion which can be drawn from the statistics is that between 1978 and 1991 the total numbers registered increased virtually fourfold. The major growth was in the areas of sexual abuse and physical neglect. It is significant that the sexual abuse figures proportionately declined from 1988 to 1991 following events in Cleveland. Clearly, the impact of the crisis dented the profession's confidence in its ability to respond to cases of suspected child sexual abuse, but also, because of the need to reframe the referral in terms of legal evidence and the significant raising of the threshold for identifying a case of sexual abuse, this resulted in fewer cases being registerable.

The largest growth between 1978 and 1991 was the catch-all 'grave concern', previously 'at risk' category. This fell rapidly between 1991 and 1992 and has had an impact on both the overall total and the relative distribution among the other categories. This decline followed the publication of *Working Together under the Children Act 1989* (1991), which recommended that the category of 'grave concern' should be discarded. These figures give an indication of the growth in public and professional awareness of child protection cases and the actual and potential amount of work involved.

Third, the extended definition and the increase in awareness and the resulting increase in referrals took place within a situation where social workers and others had a responsibility to safeguard children in the family, while at the same time safeguarding parental responsibility and ensuring that family autonomy was not thwarted. This view of protection contains within it the protection of the child but also the protection of parents and family privacy from unjustified state interventions. As previously discussed, this homogeneous view of the family which ignores the politics of gender in effect has meant the protection of some men from confronting their abusive behaviour to women and children in the family.

Fourth, these developments have been taking place in an economic and social environment which had a direct impact on Social Services Departments and social-work practice with children and families. The level of need, and therefore potential clients, grew as increasing sections of the population became marginalised from the mainstream of the economy.

A National Children's Home study (1991) showed that one in ten children under the age of 5 from families receiving a low income did not have enough to eat at least once a month because parents could not afford to buy food, while one in five of the parents, themselves, did not have food on a regular basis because of a lack of money. All the 254 families with children in the study had an unhealthy diet, not through ignorance of what constituted healthy eating but because of a lack of finance.

During this period there have also been severe limits on the resources available to other state welfare agencies. The changes in social security and the introduction of the social fund (Becker and Silburn, 1990; Berthoud, 1990), together with the harsh restrictions on 16–18-year-olds receiving benefit, have had a significant impact on children and families. Additionally, the substantial cut-back in council housing has led to increases in homelessness and households experiencing overcrowding. As a result there has been an increased potential need among children and families and therefore demands upon Social Services Departments. It is, however, apparent that Social Services Departments have not had the resources available to meet this vastly increased potential need at a time when local authorities, and other agencies, face new responsibilities (Health Committee Second Report, 1991; Schorr, 1992).

Finally, as the social-work profession has become more regulated as a way of meeting all these new demands, central government has accelerated the process of shifting resources and changing attitudes in the profession away from 'service-orientated' professional practice to a more 'business-like' organisational culture. Although it has been unable to do this directly as in the Health Service, the creation of the Audit Commission in 1983 and the re-organisation of the Social Service Inspectorate in 1985 have specifically promoted government concepts of entrepreneurial management to Social Service Departments (see Clarke, Chapter 3 of this volume). With the redefinition of the social-work role away from 'therapeutic casework', the role of the manager has changed, from an expert and consultant on skills and methods of working with clients, to a designer and monitor of systems, within which an increasing number of professional agencies are working.

The culture and gender of the new welfare manager is predominantly male, white and middle class. This may be coincidental, but studies have shown that women in senior managerial positions hold different views on their roles and responsibilities from those of male counterparts and are more likely than male managers to remain committed to the 'service ideal'. Furthermore, where men may prefer the bureaucratic aspects of their work, women managers accentuate the aspects of their employment which are supportive and caring (Eley, 1987; Cooper and Davidson, 1982).

It is important to guard against making stereotypical assumptions concerning gender roles in management but we must also avoid an explicitly masculinised culture within which women may find it increasingly difficult to work. There is a danger, therefore, that the bureaucratisation of child protection is leading to a predominantly white, male, middle-class managerial culture that is increasingly defining both the problems and solutions to the issues of child abuse in a gendered way. There is a significant danger that while this happens the experience, knowledge and skills of women practitioners become displaced.

The growth in demand in the context of reduced, or at best, barely maintained resources means that Social Services Departments are finding it increasingly difficult to develop the more wide ranging preventive family support strategies included in the Children Act 1989. Priorities and choices are being made, between the more conventional child welfare responsibilities and responding to child abuse, and choices and priorities in relation to child abuse itself. It is in this respect that the assessment of 'high risk' takes on its particular significance and reaches the centre of what it is to be professionally involved in child protection work. The task then becomes one of distinguishing the 'high risk' from the rest, so that children can be protected, parental rights and responsibilities can be safeguarded and scant resources steered to where they are likely to be the most effective.

Resources, knowledge and experience are therefore focused on assessing and sifting out 'high risk', particularly when 'high risk' cannot be unquestionably distinguished (London Borough of Brent, 1985: 289). When there is inadequate evidence to show that the situation is safe, a programme of observation and monitoring takes on essential significance. Attention is now concentrated on assessing forensic evidence so that policy and practice, while crucially dependent upon professional judgement are shaped in terms of legalism.

SHIFTING PARADIGMS OF INTERVENTION IN CHILD PROTECTION AND THE BUREAUCRATISATION OF SOCIAL WORK WITH CHILDREN AND THEIR FAMILIES

David Howe (1994) points out that the consequence of this public examination of the role of social work is that the focus of attention in social work has changed to a concentration on the 'act' rather than the 'actor'. Social-work practitioners are no longer looking for change through insight. There is now a concentration on agreements, task completion and skills training instead of therapeutic interventions.

It may have been the succession of child abuse enquiries and high media criticism that brought into doubt the ability of social workers to change those who abuse children and so be able to protect children. If it is the view of the society, government and to some degree the profession itself that imparting insight leading to change does not protect children, then what the client does rather than why he or she does it is the route along which certainty can be installed. This change in theoretical outlook is essentially adjusting the way social workers view, approach and work with clients.

Clients are now not categorised as cases but instead are called 'consumers', 'service users' and 'contractors'. Practice takes place at the level of the 'performance' and not the 'performer'. Social workers are now responding to the 'surface' of events and ignoring, or having no time or encouragement to explore, the 'depth' of people's lives and problems in a therapeutic relationship.

The dangers inherent in the social worker as technician following a practice and legal handbook can be summarised by Howe's view that

> once practice ceases to puzzle over the whys and wherefores of human behaviour, social workers no longer need to employ theories of the personality, the relationship and the social order. The social worker's practices are more likely to be task-orientated and performance related, quantifiable and measurable, product minded and subject to quality control.
>
> (Howe, 1994)

In effect, the social world of the client with its intricacies and messiness is being reduced to that of a commodity. Social work with children and their families illustrates this with the move away from enhancing children's welfare by re-educating poorly functioning families in order to protect children by recognising potentially dangerous parents.

Hudson (1992) has pointed how agencies have become pre-occupied with procedures and guidelines as a means of protecting its professionals from acknowledging and subsequently responding to the scale of the emotional and political meaning of sexual abuse. Although following procedures allows workers to feel easier about the work they do, these new 'surface' methods of predicting which children will be abused are inherently unreliable. Check-lists and risk factors are not by themselves able to protect children. Empirical studies which examine child protection practices and decision-making show how these various tensions and ambiguities are reflected in practice and the resulting consequences for children and families.

Gary Denman and David Thorpe's study (1993) examined 100 child protection cases from the point of initial allegation in a Welsh local authority for a period of nine months. Over half of the child abuse allegations were not substantiated after investigation. It is clear that a considerable amount of professional time and resources were put into this sifting process. The researchers point out that allegations of neglect are the least likely to be substantiated and the least likely to receive ongoing social work input.

Similar results are evident in a much larger study on the operations of child protection registers (Gibbons, et al., 1993). The authors concluded that about six out of every seven children who entered the child protection system at referral stage were filtered out without needing to be subjected to the child protection register. Of those actually investigated 44 per cent led to no actions at all. In only 4% of all the referred cases were children taken from home following a court order during the investigation. This is a quite a different representation of social-work practice from that depicted in Cleveland and Orkney. The more one is distanced from forensic evidential concerns the more likely it is that interventions will not take place. In 65 per cent of the neglect referrals (392 in total), the researchers could not identify any protection plans which resulted in a supportive service. Yet these children had the highest number of poverty indicators and just as many indicators of vulnerability as those referred for physical abuse or sexual abuse. Thus the repeated scenario was of children not reaching the threshold for child protection intervention, but not getting any preventive assistance either. The fact that increasing numbers of children and their families are experiencing child protection investigations to little effect is also the finding of the recent Audit Commission report, *Seen but Not Heard* (HMSO, 1994).

Local authorities have been criticised for concentrating resources at the sharp end of child protection work and not therefore fulfilling their responsibilities towards other children in need as defined under Section 17 of the Children Act. The Children Act 1993 report noted that implementation of Section 17 had been sluggish: 'Some authorities are finding it difficult to move from a reactive social policing role to a more proactive partnership approach' (DoH, 1994). The Department of Health has expressed the concern that Social Services Departments are focusing on the particular incident of abuse and losing sight of the overall welfare of the child. As a result many children are experiencing investigations without care plans unless the child's name is placed on the child protection register. Too many people are experiencing the child protection system who could possibly be more effectively assisted under the family support provision of the Act. It is not consistent with the Children Act philosophy for the gateway to family support services to be closed until the problem is presented in terms of child protection and clearly misrepresents the nature of need presented to Social Services Departments (Sone, 1994).

CONCLUSIONS

This chapter has attempted to explore the decisive factors that have led to the position we are in today with regard to social work with children and their families. It has postulated that this practice is gradually being isolated from its traditional skills base and is becoming more regulated and technical. The rise of ideals of the 'new (mainly male) managerialism', and the bureaucratisation of the service, have led to the discourse concerning child protection being reframed more and more by legal and administrative requirements and away from the concerns of predominantly female practitioners.

It could be argued that this would not matter too much if the new emphasis on child protection was producing a service that was both equitable and helpful to children and their families while affording children protection from abuse. However, the studies by Denman and Thorpe (1993), Gibbons, *et al.*, (1993) and the Audit Commission Report (1994), present a different scenario. Their results illustrate the way that processes and concerns are structured and weighted in importance and the consequences these have for the children, parents and professionals involved. The majority of cases are closed, and no further action taken early in the process. Those not subjected to registration receive little monitoring, and the children and families involved receive *little or no practical or professional assistance*. This is the consequence of child protection policy and practice which is set up essentially to identify actual or potential significant harm or high-risk situations. Repeatedly, such referrals are considered according to legalistic criteria where the assessment and identification of forensic evidence is crucial even when the allegation is not strictly provable. If referrals cannot be constructed according to these legalistic criteria, or where the allegation is not substantiated, the referral leaves the child protection system. While it must be acknowledged that allegations of abuse may be unfounded, many of the situations may well contain a number of observed anxieties and concerns but may not warrant continuing involvement under the authority of current child protection procedures.

This is a very different scenario from the more welfare-orientated social work imagined in child care in the 1950s and 1960s, and different in significance from the sections of the Children Act 1989 which stress the need for supplying practical help and support services to families and where the 'welfare of the child' is paramount. This is not to suggest that the belief in partnership and trying to consider the interests and wishes of the child are not viewed as important, but that they are crucially viewed in legalistic child protection policies and practices which are principally interested with the assessment of high risk and therefore the weighing and consideration of forensic evidence.

Events in Cleveland have illustrated the way that the framing of the particular problem leads to a set of prescribed and specific results; namely, the upholding of male authority in families at the expense of protecting children. Although the public debate that has shaped policies has been about the veracity and admissibility of children's and medical evidence, the fundamental questions concerning sexual abuse have remained unaddressed, with children not being protected as a result. Unless a better balance can be achieved between 'surface and depth' explanations and practice, social work in local authorities will not be able to protect children effectively; women practitioners will be further marginalised and isolated; and the services to children and their families will fragment further, with the private and voluntary sector offering the 'depth' and the local authority agency the 'surface'.

ACKNOWLEDGEMENTS

To Nigel Parton for his friendship and professional generosity and to John Griffith for his advice and suggestions on a previous draft.

Chapter 10

Regulation for radicals

The state, CCETSW and the academy

David Webb

There's nothing more guaranteed to excite the sociologist than the opportunity to uncover the gap between humanity's good intentions and prosaic reality. Exposing and then disposing of idealist illusions in the face of materiality remains a staple analytical device of sociology, despite the rather breathless rehabilitation of human agency in the discipline's explanatory repertoire. And what better subject on which to try out this debunking tactic than anything to do with the welfare state and those that work within it. Here we have charitable, doubtless well-intentioned and often reformist sentiment, individuals too who frequently possess the noblest of attitude and who look to serious changes in the way society ought to be organised. Yet what is the picture portrayed by those who are sociologists or who have come under their influence? That the welfare state is fiscally dependent on capitalism, thereby making a sham of anything but the most modest and conditional transformations; that welfare practitioners engage in practices that routinise cases in order to process them more readily; that these same welfare workers are reproducing social relations and transmitting ideology or, as the Foucauldians have it, are 'distributing norms'; that they support racist and sexist practices; that the 'helping' organisations within which they work are patriarchal and oppressive of disadvantaged women employees. Although claims made in the past – such as social work being what Halmos (1965) called 'altruism under social auspices' – seem endangered and naïve when set within a sociological framing of social work which casts it as politically compromised and morally suspect, it would be wrong to assume that the same scepticism should not be brought to bear upon contemporary and equivalent claims for ethical perfection.

More recently, social work (like social welfare more generally) has been pictured as swept along by post-Fordist shifts in the nature of production and underpinning work tasks, as the organisation of welfare begins to emulate that found in other spheres of the economy (Burrows and Loader, 1994). Decentralisation, team-based work, purchaser–provider quasi-markets; the decomposition of social work as a coherent (if semi-)profession in the face of a prospective independence of probation training, and signs of indivisibility between certain social-work and community nursing tasks, all suggest that something quite significant is happening to the roles and tasks of the social worker. And as sociology has charted the admittedly contested onset of postmodernity, so too has social work been set within this putative rupture in how we approach truth, reason and culture. In short, and not surprisingly, we are told that social work simply cannot stand alone and outside capitalism, trying somehow to have both its cake and eat it by existing simultaneously within and against the state. Indeed, if anything, social work is 'overdetermined' by that economic and social formation so that its status is best seen as relatively subordinate rather than as relatively autonomous. Put at its most uncompromisingly straightforward, state welfare is an element within the state apparatus, and as such will be to some extent articulated with it at both ideological and material levels. While it would be too teleological or 'functionalist' to 'read off' the nature of social work from the nature of the state, at the same time it does not take any special sociological insight to realise that the relationship between the two is worthy of reflection as we try to understand the nature of social work under conditions of contemporary change.

What passes for social work is the product of the varying capacity of certain institutions and agencies to give it a particular definition, to shape what it is that constitutes legitimate professional knowledge and the manner in which the delivery of services should be organised. In both respects this means that the nature of social work is an *accomplishment*, a construction, or the product of what Althusser called 'ideological practices'. In view of the role that social work plays in remoralising the poor, or in returning people to utility, or in policing the boundaries between waywardness and righteousness, then it is understandable that a great deal of political interest will be shown in the manner by which these duties are discharged by welfare professionals.

All this is but a continuation of that sociological worrying about how things are not as they seem, and that in our enquiries we need

to search endlessly for better (or perhaps more adequate) understandings of what is 'really' going on. It is this which allows
sociology (or at least certain traditions within the discipline) to claim
that it is a science. In truth, sociology cannot long stay with
description alone nor with the purely empirical. It is weak in resisting
the temptation to explain, to generate causal explanations, to put this
or that institution or event sequentially and conceptually before
another so that some order can be imposed on experience. It is
something that David Matza (1964) some time ago called 'soft
determinism' and which has had a contemporary echo in Giddens'
theory of structuration, whereby there is an attempt to cope with the
sheer limiting materiality of human existence without succumbing
to anti-humanist determinism. Although this shies away from reducing human activity to the remorseless and invariant force of
social circumstance, permitting instead some latitude for what is
sometimes termed 'action' or what Giddens terms 'agency', there
remains the sociological equivalent of the *deus ex machina* – the
looming presence of causal antecedents, of structure, of materiality,
or of inescapable 'social facts'.

OFSWET – THE OFFICE OF SOCIAL WORK EDUCATION AND TRAINING: A NEW NAME FOR CCETSW?

Of course social work is caught up in a wider trajectory than a history
of its own making. Its form under what is sometimes called
'postmodernity' is clearly what exercises much of this book, reflecting previous concerns to locate socially within this meta-narrative
the reasons for certain shifts in the *practices* and discourses within
which the enterprise may sit (Parton, 1994a; Howe, 1994). This
particular chapter is only obliquely about the *practice* of social work
and the various changes to the organisation of welfare agencies or
the typical work tasks of individual practitioners. Rather, it continues
an earlier attempt to say something about the role of a particular 'key
definer' of what passes for the nature of social work (Webb,1991).
Howard Becker used the notion of a 'moral entrepreneur' to capture
the motivations and interests of those competing to secure the right
to declare the boundary between virtue and waywardness. Here the
accumulation and investment of cultural and moral capital is being
managed by the statutory body responsible for the education and
training of social workers as it seeks to define the nature and scope

of competent practice and professional ethics. The Central Council for Education and Training in Social Work (CCETSW) has always done this since it was established by statute in 1971 'to promote training in relevant social work for staff in local authorities, health and social services boards in Northern Ireland, the probation service, the education welfare service and the voluntary and private sectors' (CCETSW, 1994b: 7). CCETSW sets down the content and standards of training programmes and therefore determines what it is that a proficient social worker needs to know and do. It has also an inspection role by which the Council supervises training pro- grammes in order to assure quality, something which gives it licence to lay down expectations of those universities that are associated with professional education, a point of some significance for a 'regulator' and one that will be given more attention later in this chapter.

It goes without saying that the role of CCETSW as a legitimator and definer of social-work knowledge and skills is not the product of a genteel debate among the good and the wise about what it would be nice to see in qualifying training for social work, though there is a suspicion that in CCETSW's past this may indeed have been the case. The Council has become increasingly answerable to govern- ment as an instrument for policy control over skill mix and the workforce superintendence that accompanies placing social-work training under the auspices of employers (Jones, 1989, 1994; Webb, 1992). And CCETSW with its Chair and up to 25 members appointed by the Secretary of State is nothing if not an extension of employer interests.

There have occurred a number of recent modifications to the requirements made of those centres providing social-work training and education, and it is with these and what they express about the social location of social work that this chapter is concerned. In large measure the exemplification of change is to be traced through CCETSW's Paper 30, the document that ushered in the new Diploma in Social Work (DipSW), setting down expectations and regulations about the key themes of training, morality and partnership, around which this chapter will range. Although this document has been reviewed and although there look to be revisions to the training regulations, the underlying form of the Council's strategy remains largely unaltered. There is, however, a particularly significant textual amendment which has attracted some attention. The original Paper 30 spoke about the basis for one particular aspect of its moral thrust as resting on the 'endemic racism' in British society. Not surprisingly, this was not well received in certain quarters of the administration and alone probably accounts for why CCETSW has been required to revise something which was only launched two years before this DipSW review was announced. Needless to say, the inflammatory (though empirically verifiable) utterance no longer appears in the new documentation that CCETSW has produced, accompanied no doubt by murmuring about the hubris being visited on the Council.

The revisions to Paper 30 notwithstanding, its initial appearance marked a paradigmatic shift in the discursive practice of social-work education and training. These cultural and ideological changes in the preferred content of social-work education are ones that I will try to assess as having properties that are *postmodern*. There is at the same time an equally interesting move in the way that skills and competencies are being reconstituted by CCETSW that has a distinctly post-Fordist air of workforce flexibility about it. Analytically, these general and conceptual points can be approached through seeing the Central Council as seeking to frame social work within three extremely significant and inter-linked domains: first, the stipulation of practice competence by means of a discourse around 'training'; second, the requirement of demonstrable moral conduct towards social oppression; and third, through the insistence on 'partnership' in delivering social work there is the de-centring of the academy as the site within which what passes for social work knowledge is set.

STRATEGIC CHOICE, SETTLING SCORES AND CCETSW'S SURVIVAL

Regulation occupies an important place in the analysis of modernity. Its role is in securing essential predictability for the control of productive forces and for the surveillance of the social relations which flow from these forces and upon which they depend. The panopticon was regarded by Foucault as exemplifying proximate hierarchical surveillance operating through concrete and empirical solutions to the problem of order, whereas the emergence of social control by the moral and psychological reconstruction of a person through the benign interventions of the psy-experts presents the regulation of actual or potential deviants in a 'new' form – and one that is in some way postmodern. However, neither Foucault nor

Donzelot speculates on what happens if the norm distributing agencies fail in their objective of what in an earlier epoch was called (by the Victorians – rather presciently) 'gentling the masses'. Foucault, for example, seems to consider only a progressive and unilinear trajectory of increasing complexity and sophistication as remote surveillance triumphs over proximate control. However – and Parton (1994a) alludes to this exhaustion, or crisis, of tutelage – the predicament within the welfare approach to social disruption does not automatically lead to the perfection of yet more efficient and subtle techniques of norm distribution. It leads instead to techniques of *behavioural* change, a backtracking to the future with practices involving hierarchical surveillance and more or less unmediated regulation. What we are presently witnessing (in social-work education as in social work itself) is an instance of conservative modernisation, in which economic liberalisation joins with increasingly desperate measures brought to bear in order to secure compliance with political and economic objectives.

Whilst a political and moral endorsement of the 'social' (and its psy-experts) exemplifies high modernity in securing conformity through self-regulation or by the legitimate interventions of the 'secular priests' in the resolution of personal malfunction, this inevitably depends on some sort of concordat between the state and these 'distributors of norms'. But if this breaks down, the issue of governance becomes critical. And indisputably it has broken down in the case of social work and how its training is conducted. The 'fragile discursive practice' (Parton, 1994a) of social-work education is once more under further investigation for its failure to deliver reliability of product. The evidence is clear: yet another 'functional analysis' of the roles and tasks of the social worker in order to find out exactly what it is these unreliable, if not treacherous, welfare workers actually do (Jones, 1994); and, as we have already seen, there is a politically inspired review of the DipSW almost before its first award-holders have hit the streets, as well as a Home Office 'scrutiny' of probation training with the transparent objective of recovering control of what was relinquished in the heady days of generic training in the mid-1960s. Something appears to be on the verge of a break-up: there are signs in these events of the decomposition of old certainties, with difference, fragmentation and hyper-pluralism becoming increasingly the postmodern world within which social work struggles to survive.

Despite the value-talk centred on anti-oppression – which not only cynics see as having been offered as a strategic concession to some of its constituents (Dominelli, 1991) – CCETSW exists as a quasi non-governmental regulatory body that operates only with the permission of the departments of state which sponsor and fund it. It is an element in governance that constitutes or constructs the way in which social-work education is formed and the practices and knowledge that are permissible therein. Within a context of the problematic superintendence of what the Victorians called the dangerous and threatening aggregates, social workers need to become reliable state agents and CCETSW must perforce play its part in ensuring precisely this. The recent, and as we have seen, the continuing history of the organisation revolves around its struggle to secure sufficient credibility to remain in sponsored existence. Though this context constitutes an environment which significantly shapes the possibilities that CCETSW is able to mobilise, measures taken by its senior executives within this set of imperatives should still be seen as conscious designs on how to secure the organisation's future. It is in this sense that we can use the notion of strategic choice that has played a part in the study of organisational behaviour (Bryman, 1993).

A current means of meeting the goal of corporate survival is to emulate the neo-liberal regulatory machinery that government has employed to police the activities of organisations which have been freed from the shackles of corporatism. Managing the productive forces within contemporary capitalism is set within this seeming paradox of organisational decentralisation on the one hand and centralised strategic control on the other (Hoggett, 1994). But it is only an *apparent* paradox, for there is a seamlessness to the apparatuses that play a complementary role in the maintenance of order, with the present arrangements for the administration and superintendence of social-work education serving as something of a case study of these new forms of integrated and multi-level social control. These strategies of intervention work through those three interlinked domains of training, morality and partnership that have already been identified as the new frame for social-work education. The remainder of this chapter is concerned with isolating each of these elements in turn.

TRAINING, COMPETENCIES AND PERFORMANCE

The emphasis on training and the specification of competencies has set a tightness to CCETSW's regulatory project since it allows an intrusiveness into the academy that was hitherto not possible. Up until the introduction of the new Diploma in Social Work the training requirements for professional education were relatively permissive and accordingly gave scope for a greater emphasis on knowledge than on skills. This had given the universities and colleges sufficient space to determine matters in their own light and to write the curriculum according to agendas that were only partly determined by the concerns of narrow technical proficiency. There can be little doubt that the expansion in the social sciences of the late 1960s – and sociology and more latterly 'critical' social policy exemplified this – led to a major shift in the prevailing conceptual framework through which social-work knowledge was transmitted (Jones, 1994). It seemed that control of professional socialisation had been ceded to most unreliable custodians. The independence of the academy posed an increasing problem for CCETSW, as the universities' claim for academic freedom led to doubts about the Council's capacity to give direction to training that was not going to be compromised by the mischievous meddling of people for whom academic values had supplanted professional ones. Quite simply this meant that it would never be possible for CCETSW to exercise leverage (and thereby secure its own future) unless that autonomy could be broken.

From the early 1970s onwards there has been a frequently articulated – and more often than not politically orchestrated – set of public utterances doubting the calibre of social workers, with various strategies of shaming, mockery and degradation being brought to play in repudiating not only state welfare workers, but those whose social incompetence or deviance found them in the inept clutches of these 'do-gooders'. Much of the 'evidence' that something was seriously wrong with the capabilities of social workers was supplied through the increasing number of child abuse enquiries. CCETSW did not demur from this (Jones, 1989), and behind the scenes contributed to the dissemination of the view that training needed a thorough overhaul. The then professional qualification – the Certificate of Qualification in Social Work (CQSW) was portrayed by CCETSW itself as inadequate as a basis for contemporary practice as it sought to show government how it would put the world of training to right. Key (if maverick) opinion-formers within the academy such as Martin Davies (Professor of Social Work at the University of East Anglia) and Robert Pinker (of the London School of Economics) also played a significant role in the framing of this challenge to standards in social-work education, largely from a sociological 'logic-of-place' perspective which owed a good deal to structural-functionalism. Attacking both the excesses of ambitious (often politically radical) social-work-driven meta-narratives of social change as well as the corporatist interferences of CCETSW in the academy, these neo-liberal voices added to the increasing destabilisation of the enterprise of social-work education.

As so often, a moment of crisis coincides with, or prompts, changes in personnel. In 1986, a new director was appointed to CCETSW. Quite clearly he was charged with putting matters straight and with mounting something of a last ditch attempt to show that CCETSW had a future. Central to this would have to be the delivery of an improved social-work training. It was an initiative that required various endorsements, although at that particular moment of supreme confidence within the Thatcher administration there was little inclination to be forthcoming except for the most hawkish of developments. The answer for CCETSW to this problem of providing sufficient robustness, and the key to government support, was the employer-led initiatives that were taking place in vocational education more widely and which were (and still are) guided by the National Council for Vocational Qualifications. CCETSW promoted very actively employer involvement in the various designs for the new award that it laid out, principally on the grounds that education had become so deficient that the only way that universities and colleges could remedy these failings (for which they were represented as accountable) was at long last to heed the voice of the 'consumer'.

It was clear that 'collaboration' (or the rather more palatable 'partnership') was to be the linchpin of the strategy to bring the colleges into line. Part of this was the concerted promotion of the Certificate of Social Service (CSS) as equivalent to professional education, something that it had never been designed to be. This award, which had been introduced in 1977 as an in-service route for social services staff generally in residential settings, had always been set as a lower-level academic qualification to the CQSW, although there was a widespread view among employers that it produced competent workers. But its most significant distinguishing feature was the *joint management* arrangements that saw the mandatory involvement of social-work agencies in determining the nature and content of education and training. Without such involvement educational centres would not secure CCETSW's approval to operate the scheme. Despite all the evidence about the expense and the cumbersomeness of the managerial structures of CSS, it emerged in effect as the model for the future Diploma in Social Work, almost entirely because of the partnership between colleges and agencies upon which it rested. And interestingly, the CSS resonated with a strong anti-elitist sentiment in some quarters of the educational world, especially that in the further education sector which had been assiduously courted by CCETSW as it sought to build new strategic alliances that would cut across what would otherwise be an unhelpful educational unity. CSS was the Trojan horse welcomed by the academy (or at least some sections of it), from which spilled the proposals and plans for what was to become the Diploma in Social Work. CCETSW would bring the querulous secular clerics of a recalcitrant academy into line and at the same time offer a way to restructure the welfare workforce through a realignment of the training and education mix (Pinker, 1984). In this way CCETSW was an eager exemplar of social work's own post-Fordism of flexibility, decentralisation and market plurality. It 'appeared' to loosen its direct control over education, creating instead pseudo-autonomous programme providers operating as quasi-businesses founded on semi-contractual mutual partnerships in order to meet the 'specifications' set by the Council.

These moves are aspects of recent shifts in the relative weighting given to education and training within social work, and in particular the emergent emphasis on the specifying of tasks to be done rather than knowledge to be gleaned. The movement is from the depth explanations of modernism's concern with transcendent truth to postmodernity and its multiplicities of surface performance. But postmodernity is not an epoch which is beyond control: rather, it offers a vision of other modes by which control is exercised. Thus the performance of *tasks* or competencies is in the public domain, so these are capable of being owned, set and controlled to a high degree by others. They are observable and therefore verifiable and predictable. *Knowledge*, on the other hand, tends towards being more private, less open to the specification of what it should encompass. It is less calculable and more idiosyncratic: it smacks of abstraction and unreliability – you cannot know what someone is thinking, but you can see what they do. Because the regulatory discourse that CCETSW has embraced must perforce operate with certainties and the measurable, the pedagogic consequences within social-work education have followed accordingly, with the consequential de-centring of the academy.

Through this reconstruction the social-work academy has become a virtual extension of the National Council for Vocational Qualifications (Jones, 1989). Geared to, and obsessed by, the prosaic achievement of competence (and only the English could erect policy around the humdrum of competence rather than the excitement of excellence), the new approach to training produces superficially accomplished performers able to demonstrate through appearance and exhibition their entitlement to certification. The dramaturgical connotation is significant, with identity in high modernity being more and more built around the 'face work' of bearing semblance (Giddens, 1991).

Social-work education seems to have become firmly established as a surface-oriented activity: in fact the traditional Arnoldian idea of education sits ever uneasily within the enterprise as an 'old-fashioned' diversion just as does the modernising project, which is about exposing the errors and limitations of pre-scientific, partial and superstitious thought. 'Education' for all its civility and compromises with the dominant culture, wrenches the heart out of the cherished and taken-for-granted as it inspects and interrogates. Training, on the other hand, cannot be bothered with these questions of deep structure. It looks rather to the observationally verifiable. It suspends consideration of the existentially or epistemologically troubling. 'Training' takes to some sort of ultimate resolution the empiricism of English modernity because it deletes the radical and querulous refutationist elements that empiricism contained. Training leaves us with only the illusion of certainty because of what it otherwise suspends.

Training for competence therefore yokes social workers to the requirements of those who purchase their labour as professional expertise becomes increasingly commodified through the breaking of any semblance of generic unity. Through functional analysis of the social worker's job (as CCETSW is currently doing) is generated a strategy for the control both of employees and of education since the contract for delivering these becomes capable of very high degrees of precision. The fragmentation of occupational activity by the more or less exact specification of skills lends rational measurement of use value through the segmentation of those skills. Less tied to any one particular job or post, these skills can now be transferred from setting to setting, and across boundaries which were hitherto set by the restrictive practices of occupational and professional power. The initiatives in joint training between social workers and community mental health nurses stand as an instance in which labour flexibility is being facilitated through the involvement of validating bodies – which in this case includes the national boards for nursing alongside CCETSW (Webb, 1992). Functional specialism has also enabled the Home Office to begin its long-planned move to withdraw probation officer training from generic education, on the ostensible grounds that separate and specific skills are needed which can no longer be provided through the Diploma in Social Work. There is little reason not to see this as a further instance of how differentiation of task leads to fragmentation of activity and an expansion in the subordination of welfare workers to very tightly specified employer concerns (see also Pinch, 1994).

THE STYLE COUNCIL?

Parallel with the regulatory character of the new award with its highly prescriptive stipulation of competencies was a wider set of injunctions within social-work education: as we have seen, judgements of capability are increasingly set in terms of the superficial certainties that come from task specification and competencies. And this has generated an orthodoxy reflected in the new morality that is enunciated through CCETSW's declarations. This is not to enter into a foolhardy discussion about the rightness or wrongness of that discourse, but it is rather to see it as an expression of an emerging process of 'surface' competencies that must be demonstrated behaviourally. For good reason or not, the requirements that have been promulgated about anti-oppressive practice are part and parcel of the same training mentality that has pervaded the rest of the regulator's view of social-work education. Superficially radical, this approach to values none the less exists within a performance-orientated discourse which has been set within a similarly behavioural/surface mode to the other competencies that are now required to be demonstrated by the tyro social worker.

I have elsewhere offered what I called a speculation on the 'sociogenesis' of this 'new moral discourse', something which is marked by righteousness, censoriousness and certitude as well as by the preparedness to implement the sanction of ban (Webb, 1991). I called this 'puritan', arguing that the momentum within social work was encouraged by earlier modifications to the law which 'progressive' forces in the 1960s and 1970s had applauded as successful interventions in civil society around the social divisions of gender, race and childhood. But the cultural forces at work are again contrapuntal. Although there are here advances in the protection of vulnerable citizens, these changes in social solidarity expressed through the law also entail permission to renounce an earlier ethic of forgiveness which can now be replaced by one marked by the superficiality of retribution. The sinner has no hope of experiencing the abstraction or tentativeness of redemption, or of receiving philanthropy under social auspices, but is instead cast out into the community, that modern equivalent of a wilderness.

I did not in that earlier piece locate my speculations within a set of considerations that looked specifically at the features of social work in the modern age, though I think that by implication the discussion in 'Puritans and Paradigms' approached this question, for it remarked on the formal similarity between the rhetorical certainties of Thatcherism and those of the new paradigm. However, I have sought here to extend those ideas a little by taking another perspective towards this new moral discourse. CCETSW's value-talk around oppression issues is carried out within what Callinicos (1990) discusses as the abandonment of class and the de-politicising of resistance, substituting the realist categories of the social sciences with a list of oppressions jostling for attention and action. It is also divorced from any account of causation or of inter-relationships between social categories. As David Howe has noted, this expresses a postmodern preference for ontology over epistemology, where truth resides in the being of various status positions rather in elaborate systems of 'abstract' social categories such as, for example, the less resiliently experiential one of class. Truth then becomes de-centred and localised (Howe, 1994). Certainly the enunciation of those differences which have not hitherto been represented within discourses of social division constitutes a lifting of amnesia within the humanities and social sciences. Yet fragmentation around a multitude of oppressions and the politicisation of difference have a resonance with the seductive discourses of locality, community and empowerment that have figured within the rhetoric of neo-liberalism. It is difference rather than commonality that CCETSW has found itself endorsing. Ostensibly progressive, at the same time this sits within a set of cultural practices in a way which Machiavelli probably would have found commendable.

None the less, there is inherent instability within the new discourse that CCETSW has sought to establish within the value-talk of social work, demonstrating that there remains a tension between various domains of certainty and orthodoxy. As part of the most recent review of qualifying training CCETSW has been forced to withdraw the declaration about endemic racism in Britain that appears in annex 5 to the original 1991 regulations for the Diploma in Social Work (CCETSW, 1994a). Not surprisingly, given its manifest clash with sentiments about the basically decent nature of Britain, the clause had caused consternation in ministerial circles: it was clear that a new chair of Council (appointed in the summer of 1993) was set as a high priority the task of seeing the offending passage removed. Ironically, what seems to have made this victory relatively easy lies with the way in which CCETSW had effectively excluded the very social sciences (and in effect the social scientists too) that could have been brought to bear on demonstrating empirically that racism (and any other oppression for that matter) *is* indeed structurally endemic. But because CCETSW has consistently failed to acknowledge the complexities in conceptualising oppression (and in particular the analytical problems of determining system and personal attributes), it has found itself manifestly unable to mount a defence of its position. Furthermore, since its approach to anti-discrimination has been framed around competencies to the almost total exclusion of analysis and 'knowledge', it remains epistemologically unstable. By this I mean that anti-discrimination becomes precarious and easily eroded, as undoubtedly it has been for CCETSW in its capitulation to those who would seek its removal from Paper 30.

It is in this sense that CCETSW exemplifies certain features that could be regarded as quintessentially postmodern. There is the absence of a deep structure (about 'causes', for example) to the new moral discourse, which remains primarily framed within the superficiality of rhetoric and competencies. There is the excising or obscuring of complexity and a reluctance to give much space to the interconnectedness between oppressions which instead become rendered as competing, almost 'individualistic' characteristics (Graham, 1992). There is the associated imagery of oppressions being somehow choosable, arrayed almost as in a market for selection. Furthermore, CCETSW has in general given licence to a strong essentialist inclination of the kind that Robert Merton some time ago called 'insiderist' (1972), whereby the possession of certain physical attributes (gender, 'race') become not only necessary but sufficient to guarantee that the individual can convey an appropriate position on the matter at hand. As Roger Sibeon puts it after his very detailed consideration of the reductionist tendencies within the current value-talk of social work: 'essentialist theoretical categorisations that conflate . . . complex empirical realities have inevitably produced an ineffectual politics of . . . fragmentation and division' (1991). And this is precisely where CCETSW has ended up, unable to sustain a stance that it has so forcefully demanded of others. The consequences of all this for the social-work academy have not been insignificant either, as it has become caught up in the educational and moral re-alignment that has been orchestrated by the validating body.

NO DIRECTION KNOWN: DERACINATING THE ACADEMY

The activity of social-work education has been noticeably reframed, culminating in the cluster of changes associated with the Council's Paper 30. There has been the supplanting of education by training; the sequestering of discourses of depth by those of surface; the setting aside of knowledge for skills, and the general triumph and solemnising of 'competencies' over the complexities of abstraction. This is about casting anew the definition of what passes for social work as a practical and conceptual activity. It is about synchronicity winning over the diachronic.

CCETSW has established a range of regulations and requirements for the education and training of social workers, which, if the academy is to remain in the business, it has been obliged to accept. This new agenda has altered the balance of autonomy hitherto enjoyed by social-work education, and instead through 'programme partnerships' has brought it into a direct and subordinate client relationship if not with employers, then at least with the new manager cadres of the personal social services. CCETSW, for all its pronouncements about 'combating oppression' has effectively notar-ised relationships of a kind that are fully consonant with those of conservative modernisation. Its *structural* position is set four-square within what were once called the ideological state apparatuses: 'surface' exhortations to repudiate discrimination sit alongside what is in effect an endorsement of neo-liberalism.

All this is in its widest sense about an alignment to two sets of moral obligations, both of which run through the enterprise of social-work education. These concern the pursuit of truth, and its transcend-ence of other loyalties, alongside the recognition that what Merton called 'group-influenced perspectives' about social divisions have indeed contributed significantly to sensitising us to matters that rightly demand our intellectual attention (Merton, 1972: 44). Somehow there needs to be a resolution of these increasingly conflicting demands if social work is to hold a place within the academy. With the 'new direction' taken by CCETSW pushing the venture in a particular way, then it may be timely to wonder whether the interests of social-work *education* might not be best served by rethinking, perhaps quite radically, the relationship between qualifying training and the social-work academy.

IN OTHER WORDS . . .

The new Diploma in Social Work did lots of things, all of them consistent with CCETSW's stated or covert objectives. *First*, and as living expression of an anti-intellectual 'component of the national culture' (Anderson, 1968), the organisation revenged itself on the universities, who had been seen as uppity, too clever by half and unwilling to bring the sociological 'radicals' within social-work education into line. From now on the universities would be unable to move without taking into account the 'sensible' concerns of welfare agencies, something which would be guaranteed to check the indulgences of the academy. *Second*, CCETSW was able to demonstrate to government that it could deliver reliably within the prevailing NVQ-driven and employer-led ethos of vocational training. It thereby acted as a 'relay' of government policy to secure a trustworthy and predictable labour force of welfare workers whose previous unpredictability, unreliability and autonomy were seen to be the source of the ills that they should be solving (Jessop, 1994). *Third*, it served as a vehicle for integrating new and sometimes querulous entrants to social work. By virtue of the changing demographic and ideological profile of both practitioners and, increasingly, members of the academy, there was a danger that training was on the verge of meeting its own particular 'legitimation crisis'. *Fourth*, CCETSW used the new award at least to try to repair the years of indifference that it had shown to probation training and therefore to the Home Office, because it had a means to demonstrate that the needs of all branches of social work were now fully encompassed by its flexible and competency-specific model. *Fifth*, and as accumulation of the other achievements, CCETSW was able to secure its own position as an increasingly reliable agent of government and ministerial and departmental concerns.

This chapter has been an attempt to understand the way in which social workers, as 'technicians of normalisation' are constituted as agents of a particular strategy of governance via the injunctions issued through the validating body which sets the training agenda. It considered the paradox of superficial radicalism occurring within the shell of a reactionary neo-liberal state and speculated about the degree to which what I have elsewhere called the new moral discourse of social work is an expression of 'life-style' adjustments to the postmodern world that social work has come to inhabit. Above all, the chapter considered the role of CCETSW as the instrument for securing the *dirigiste* restructuring of professional training through framing professional social work as a flexible, technically specific (and highly specified) enterprise in which skill-mix considerations are put to work at the behest of employers. As part of this enterprise we saw that CCETSW has deleted the abstractions, scepticisms and meta-narratives of the social sciences in favour of surface renderings of complex social and moral dilemmas as predominantly technical difficulties. In one guise CCETSW has promulgated a set of moral axioms, while in another has contributed to the 'modernisation' of social care so that it can be contained within the framework of employer-led considerations. Seemingly progressive in the domain of surface representations around words and statements, the deeper structure of compliance and complicity with the neo-liberal state's agenda is only revealed when we suspend our infatuation with CCETSW as a disseminator of utterance but read it instead as 'an almost perfectly designed vehicle' for the implementation of the conservative modernisation of social work (Brewster, 1992).

The theme that has been pursued here is of course about the regulation of social-work education. This reflects the widespread neo-liberal practice of setting boundaries to the liberties and freedoms that have been promulgated through ideological rhetoric and organisational deregulation. Variety and local conditions may appear to empower and legitimise local consortia which 'deliver' training, but in reality the regulatory framework and the specification of competencies is doing no more than establish a national curriculum in social work. The creation of programme consortia into which have been inserted the interests if not of employers then of a new cadre of public-service managers has simply exemplified the cross-flowing features that are widespread throughout contemporary political economy. This 'dissipates and splits into a plethora of localised and partial policies pursued by local or partial interests' (Parton, 1994a: 28). So CCETSW promotes decentralisation of programme delivery while simultaneously imposing a set of requirements, regulations and monitoring obligations that significantly expand the intrusiveness of the state into the determination of the social-work curriculum. CCETSW, whatever its pronouncements about the value base of the profession, is part of the state apparatus, and to overlook this is to be seduced by the appeal of idealist postmodern utterances of limitless possibility.

Chapter 11

Anti-intellectualism and the peculiarities of British social work education

Chris Jones

This chapter seeks to shed some light on the peculiarities of British social-work education. I use the term 'peculiarities' deliberately because it is now necessary to recognise the uniqueness of professional social-work education in Britain today. It is unique in the sense that there is probably no other comparable society which has a social-work education which is so precarious, uniform and state regulated. It is precarious because there are now serious questions as to whether social-work education has a long-term future in British higher education. The educational justification for its current location in universities is being increasingly questioned as it shifts increasingly towards competencies and training outcomes. The sheer bureaucratic complexities of course management and the insecurities arising out of the short-term decisions of agencies with regard to the provision of placements are also contributing to the precariousness of professional social-work education as it currently exists. Many of these ponderous structures are directly related to the now unprecedented degree of external regulation of social-work courses, which in turn give rise to its peculiar uniformity – peculiar in the sense that the domain of social work is a deeply contested domain concerning how people live and manage their lives, survive or fail, interact with the state and one another. In many other societies this leads to diversity in social-work education, reflecting differing perspectives and positions. This is not so in Britain today.

British social-work education is also unique in its anti-intellectualism and its hostile stance to the social sciences. Since 1975 there has been an on-going process of theoretical stripping out of the social-work curriculum. In its place students are increasingly confronted with a mish-mash of methods, skills and values teaching, often lacking in any coherence. Values in particular have come to occupy a strangely central position, with CCETSW appearing to believe that they can be a substitute for knowledge and understanding. There is no comparable system of social-work education in the world which is so nationally uniform, uninspired and tailored so closely to the requirements of major state employers.

This chapter is an attempt to understand how we have arrived at this position, and argues that it is naïve to locate these current difficulties as solely the result of a New Right onslaught on welfare professionals. Rather, the chapter seeks to highlight a number of continuities in the construction and development of social-work education which have long predisposed it towards anti-intellectualism, which have made it particularly vulnerable to the recent New Right agenda of de-professional regulation. The chapter looks forward to a time when social work in Britain will take education seriously and recognise the importance of thinking; to a time when Prime Ministers don't demand less understanding and more condemnation and when to think is not considered as being dangerous.

CONTAMINATION

Social work from its modern origins in the creation in 1869 of the Charity Organisation Society (COS) has been considered an activity that risks the radical contamination of those working with the most disadvantaged groups in society (Bosanquet, 1916: 131). Just as the Colonial Office was concerned that some of its personnel might 'go native' and see the world from the standpoint of the colonised rather than the coloniser, so the same has been true of social work. The act of placing social workers, chosen and selected for their 'niceness' and compassionate outlook, in the midst of the worst excesses of poverty and hardship in society is not without its risks for authority (Jones, 1978: 189–92). This context of social-work practice has always been one which can as easily sustain a perspective that sees human suffering as a consequence of systemic inequalities rather than individual or familial pathology.

The concern to prevent social workers from being either radicalised or demoralised by their daily experience of contact and involvement with some of the most deprived and impoverished sections of society was a driving force in the creation and development of formal social-work education at the beginning of the twentieth century. This notion that a carefully constructed education programme rather than an apprenticeship training regime was essential if field workers were going to cope with the pressures of the job and be immunised from disillusionment or even radical contamination was certainly prevalent within mainstream state social work at least until the mid-1970s, when opinion began to shift decisively. Marshall gave clear expression to this concern when he wrote of the purpose of social-work education:

The primary aim here is, I think, to satisfy the personal needs of the social workers themselves, to prevent internal mental conflicts, and to answer questions which they are bound to ask and must be enabled to answer to their own satisfaction if they are to give themselves whole-heartedly to their work inspired by a sense of purpose. In this connection I should like to refer once more to MacIver's book. He points out the limitations of social work; the services offered are often only palliatives, leaving the root causes unaffected. It may even be that they perpetuate the causes by making the effects more tolerable. Yet the social worker is moved by an emotional desire to help in the creation of a better world. How can this urge be reconciled with the limitations of the daily task? And, he answers, 'The social worker must in short be socially educated, must acquire as a student of economics and sociology a background of intellectual convictions. . . . *The social worker who has no background of social philosophy is at the mercy of a thousand discouragements.*'

(1946: 16–17, emphasis added)

MAKING SOCIAL WORKERS SAFE

The imperative of 'making safe' the social worker to work in the midst of human suffering without turning into a radical social critic has been a core principle in determining the content and form of the social-work curriculum. It has also been, as this chapter seeks to illustrate, why the very concept of education within social work (and in many other occupations concerned with social regulation and reproduction) takes on a particular meaning and cannot be assumed to imply a singular attention to the pursuit of truth and understanding. It is evident, for example, from the formation of the School of Sociology by the COS in 1902, that for 'knowledge' to be selected as appropriate and relevant for inclusion in the social-work curriculum, it must generally support the *primacy* of individualisation and endorse the prevailing social order. This is not only essential to the very possibility of state social work – a possibility that had to be argued for between 1945 and 1968 (see Jones, 1978) – but essential if students were to be intellectually prepared to legitimate their intrusion into the lives of vulnerable clients. As an American social-work teacher noted, one of the key tasks of social-work education is to provide the practitioner with the confidence 'to enter intimately into the personal and social problems of others without any taint of meddling' (Smith, 1957: 2).

After the Second World War the political climate was such that social welfare interventions rooted in religious or overtly moralistic frames of reference were no longer politically acceptable. To have any form of legitimacy, the temper of the period demanded that the moral imperatives of social work should be presented in the language of scientific rationality, expertise and professionalism. This point was later recognised by a group of British social-work students who noted 'the importance of professional status as indicating a body of knowledge and degree of skill, as opposed to mere do-goodery and as a defence of one's position' (Anon, 1968, appendix B).

For social work to gain its place in the post-1945 social democratic welfare state it had to overcome its charitable legacy. For the working-class poor and the labour movement in general, charity was despised for its condescension and patronage. Among the modernising and reform-orientated elites, social work carried a not dissimilar reputation as being an essentially class-based moral activity undertaken by the worthy genteel. It was in order to overcome such legacies that the post-war leaders of British social work were committed to securing professional recognition for the activity, and this required a considerable attention to language and presentation. 'Long words' and 'abstract terms' (Deed, 1953: 305) became part of the 'professional name game' (Dillon, 1969), which as that doyenne of post-1945 British social work Eileen Younghusband so openly acknowledged, allows social work to gain respect and status while preserving its underlying, core moral perspective. Social science and research, she claimed,

> make it respectable to talk about 'factors in social pathology' instead of the undeserving poor; 'community stimulation' instead of getting lonely people to the Settlement social; 'providing positive incentives to socially acceptable behaviour' instead of helping with the Brownie Pack; 'psychopathic personalities'

instead of hopeless scroungers; 'rehabilitating the socially mal-adjusted' instead of trying to reform anyone or anything. The essential rose remains unchanged by this change of names but, if anyone is helped thereby to see more clearly, to think more deeply, to diagnose more truly and to treat more effectively, then this change and all others that succeed it are all to the good.

(Younghusband, 1951: 161–2)

This quotation reveals the specific and utilitarian manner in which the social-work establishment so often approaches the social sciences and social research. Theories, perspectives, insights and research findings are plundered and adopted to the extent that they support the prevailing tenets of the activity – the essential rose. Mainstream social work has rarely looked to the social sciences purely in a spirit of genuine intellectual enquiry or exploration, searching for new insights and understandings which might in turn lead to new forms of practice and intervention. As Wootton (1959) so clearly demonstrated, the celebrated pragmatic and eclectic approach to the construction of modern social work's knowledge base was as much concerned with gilding its reputation with a patina of scientism as it was with the pursuit of knowledge and understanding.

This generation of what Everett Hughes called 'collective preten-sion' (Hughes, 1951/71) was, in the case of social work, as much targeted internally at social workers as it was to any external audience. The seemingly never-ending perpetuation of poverty and human suffering even in societies where there are clear improve-ments in social and economic provision ensures that state social work inevitably remains a deeply contested activity. The subsequent insistence by the elites that the persistence of inequality, poverty and human suffering in the midst of plenty is ultimately located within individuals and households rather than in societal processes and institutions places acute pressures on social workers. Little wonder then that such attention is given to their preparation and socialisation.

SELECTIVE KNOWLEDGE

What little work has been done exploring and analysing social-work curricula exposes the partiality and conservatism of its core know-ledge base. For example, in their separate investigations of social work's use of sociology in the curricula, both Leonard (1966) and Heraud (1967) discovered that those aspects of sociology chosen for inclusion were those which reinforced and supported the reformist and familialist domain assumptions of social work (Leonard 1966: 22). In his analysis of social-work examination papers, Heraud similarly noted that 'sociology, to those who set the papers, is mainly concerned with questions about the family and that this is the main reason for having sociology in the course' (1967: 14). Critical material, he observed, which pointed to radically different explanations of social problems was notably absent – 'there was a lack of concern with the whole field of social control '(p. 15) – and '[the] overall perspective was eclectic and functionalist' (p. 16). Descriptive accounts of malfunctioning families and communities predominated over analysis.

Analytical and critical texts from sociology and social policy were not only excluded or marginalised on many British social-work courses during the 1950s and 1960s, but both of these disciplines became increasingly subordinated to varieties of Freudian psychology. Psychoanalysis – or at least a partial version, as we discuss below – provided social work in those years with a semblance of theoretical coherence which it has never since regained. Its advantages have been well documented (Yelloly, 1975; Britton, 1954; Irvine, 1956). It allowed social work to claim a legitimating knowledge base which resonated with the principal concerns of social democratic social reform by affirming the possibility that everyone was capable of achieving citizenship. In this it broke distinctively with the earlier biological thrust of much theorising on poverty and inequality which claimed that the undeserving poor and destitute were eugenically unfit and biologically incapable of being rehabilitated. This in turn supported and legitimated many of the authoritarian and punitive policies which typified the state's response to marginal and surplus populations from the middle of the nineteenth century up until the outbreak of the Second World War. The embrace of Freudian perspectives was critical to the transformation of social work. After 1945 social work was increasingly sponsored by the state to work specifically with those sections of the poor and destitute who had previously been categorised as irredeemable/unhelpable. Psychoanalytic ideas were a crucial factor in this transformation.

PSYCHO-ANALYTICAL RESPECTABILITY

Notwithstanding the humanitarian and progressive potential of ideas which supported a notion that every human being irrespective of their social condition and status could be included in the body politic, psychoanalysis provided social work with much-needed scientific credibility to assert its value and place within the emerging framework of social democratic reforms (Bailey and Brake, 1975: 6). It contributed to a raft of arrogant claims between 1948 and 1968. The many government reports of those years which saw the scope and range of social work extended contained remarkable claims about the value of social work. Not only was social work presented as a cheap alternative to expensive residential and institutional care but it was also claimed that a body of trained social workers could rid society of the problems of self-perpetuating poverty among the renamed residuum – problem families; that the scourge of juvenile delinquency now re-presented as a symptom of inadequate socialisation, especially mothering, could be cured by the interventions of social workers providing the parenting and role models of which boys in particular had been apparently deprived. Psychoanalysis legitimised and re-invigorated casework and, if not actually practised with clients, it allowed the occupation to make fervent claims for professional recognition on the basis that its interventions and methods were informed by science rather than moral whim or predisposition (Lubove 1966: 610).

Despite the potential and value of Freudian ideas, especially their importance in pushing back the claims of biologism with its fascistic connotations when it came to managing marginalised and surplus sections of the population, mainstream social work was never less than carefully selective in its embrace of psychoanalysis. Those elements which focused on familial relationships, maturation and the unconscious were seized upon and, as Pearson (1975) argued, bowdlerised. Freud's and subsequent neo-Freudian work which looked at the inter-relationship of social structure and process and its impact on people was generally ignored. The work of Marcuse, for example, which was so influential in the late 1960s combining as it did Marxist and Freudian perspectives rarely featured on the reading lists of social-work teachers. Instead, social-work intellectuals and writers drew only on those parts of the Freudian tradition which reinforced long-running themes of personal and familial pathology as being at the root of social problems.

Although there is much within psychoanalysis which can contribute to the possibilities of progressive and humane social work it is somewhat paradoxical to note that this 'caring profession' tended to draw on Freudian ideas to construct an image of clients as 'greedy demanding children, always clamouring for material help, always complaining of unfair treatment or deprivation; this attitude shades into paranoid imagining' (Irvine, 1954: 27). In a survey of Social Services Departments twenty years later, Satyamurti observed that

> the language that social workers use about their clients, often jokingly, seems often still to be based on an image of them as good or naughty children. . . . It seemed, too, that when social workers referred to a 'difficult case' they did not mean that the client presented problems that were difficult to solve, but that he was demanding and time consuming as a difficult child.
>
> (1974: 9)

It is a somewhat sobering experience analysing social-work education and its knowledge base. For, in its mainstream at least, historical exploration of the past 100 years reveals startling continuities, such as social work's construction of clients as generally unworthy and manipulative individuals. Such a construction has contributed to a tragic legacy whereby clients are too often disregarded, not listened to and generally presented as people who don't count. This in turn must contribute to the episodes of cruelty and inhumanity which are periodically exposed, ranging from pindown in Staffordshire to Frank Beck in Leicestershire (see Wardhaugh and Wilding, 1993). One cannot but wonder about the impact of mainstream social work's construction of clients on this 'writing off' of vulnerable people.

THE DEMISE OF THE PSYCHO-ANALYTIC PARADIGM IN SOCIAL WORK

The collapse in the influence of psychoanalysis on social-work education and practice was a decisive moment in the changing fortunes of British social-work education. Its demise was due to a range of pressures which followed from the creation of unified personal social services bureaucracies in the early 1970s. Soon after, the fiscal crisis of the local state, which was to run from 1976 right through the 1980s and beyond, accelerated the process of change set in motion by re-organisation. It was deeply ironic for social work that the achievement of its much sought-after goal to be organised and unified in a single state agency under its professional control and direction (and not under medicine, which had dominated social work for much of the post-1945 period) should so rapidly turn into a nightmare. As early as 1974 the newly formed local authority Social Services Departments were being described by some influential voices within social-work education as inhospitable environments for the practice of social work (Goldberg, 1974: 268). Not only were social-work practitioners having to confront the new working environment of large, impersonal bureaucracies with their extended command structures, but they were also discovering that the bombardment of referrals was not coming from clients directly but rather from an array of state and public authorities which were exploiting the formation of a single agency to off-load their problematic and time-consuming tenants/pupils/patients/claimants/debtors and so forth. The rising caseloads and the new demands of the bureaucracy on practitioners all contributed to create a work situation whereby it was becoming increasingly impossible to undertake casework, at least in the manner informed by the psychoanalytical paradigm. After all, this social work method demands time, given its emphasis on the therapeutic relationship between social worker and client. It also requires some cooperation from the client. On both counts this was proving increasingly difficult.

The impact of the fiscal crisis and the consequent demands of the IMF that social expenditure should be significantly curtailed was particularly damaging for state social work so soon after the formation of the Social Services Departments (SSDs). Despite some early budgetary protection (NALGO, 1989), SSDs were under growing financial pressure, unable to meet either the demands of an increasing elderly population or the casualties of mounting unemployment and growing poverty. Even before the election of Margaret Thatcher in 1979, these pressures were leading to the first fissures in the social democratic consensus which had shaped social welfare expansion and development in Britain since the Second World War. At the very least, managers were being pressed to deliver 'value for money' and run their services according to the dictates of accountancy rather than more nebulous ideals of public service. Moreover, now that secure and moderately waged career structures were available within state social work, there was a greater influx of men, many of whom enjoyed rapid managerial promotion (as against women). The re-gendering of social work, especially with respect to its senior management was, as Foster (1991) has pointed out, a significant force in the emergent managerialism of the organisation and delivery of social-work services. None of these developments constituted a conducive framework for casework in its classical mould where outcomes and effectiveness were not easily measured, at least by the preferred tools of accountancy.

RADICAL IMPULSES

Simultaneously, as social policy was tilting rightwards, social-work practice and in particular professional education was feeling the impact of the radical and critical currents which pulsed through many Western societies during the late 1960s and early 1970s. The expansion of higher education with the creation of the polytechnics, followed by the growth of state social work as a result of the Seebohm re-organisations, saw many of the new social science graduates drawn into and attracted by social-work careers. Many of these new recruits posed a challenge to social-work courses and the academy. Often inspired by the social movements of the times, including a resurgent feminism, the new entrants to the profession increasingly questioned and rejected the established individualised tenets of social work. Their previous education, especially in the case of social science graduates, had, in many instances, exposed them to emerging radical insights in a range of social science disciplines including philosophy, sociology, social policy and psychology. Despite the diversity of disciplines there was a common strand of challenging traditional authority and its concomitant 'truths'. In key social policy texts poverty was beginning to be seen once more as a systemic feature of capitalist societies rather than some moral malfunction of specific problem families; in critical social psychology texts such as those written by Laing, Cooper and Marcuse and in a range of feminist texts the sanctity of the patriarchal family was being seriously questioned; the 'new' deviancy theorists were posing penetrating questions about the nature of deviance and were re-focusing on the state and state professionals such as social workers and probation officers as being implicated in the reproduction of deviance. The domain assumption of mainstream social work that society, despite some imperfections, was essentially structured and concerned with the welfare of all its citizens was, from all these diverse quarters, being systematically challenged. Normality, for example, was being exposed as a partial social construction in the interests of the elites at the expense of the majority. Such developments were not peculiar to Britain. New and difficult questions were being asked and considered by many young people; questions which in many cases were particularly threatening to traditional social work. In the case of British social work it was particularly problematic as the changes in practice noted earlier were simultaneously undermining the occupation's confidence and certainty. The result of all these processes and changes was such that, as Katherine Kendall noted at the time: 'schools of social work throughout the world are passing through a period of intense pre-occupation with the purpose of social work in society . . . social work education is in trouble in its essence and on its boundaries' (1972: 6). Within the British context, the combination of the expansion of state social work, the concomitant collapse in the legitimacy of casework as both knowledge base and method, the emergence of younger social-work students more prone to be vociferous and critical, proved to be a particularly dramatic cocktail. A brief review of curricula at that time reveals that many courses abandoned their previous psychoanalytical core and retreated into systems theory or a more general eclecticism (Jones, 1978). Some courses, for example, seemed to take the view that it was better not to take any particular theoretical stand at all but allow a free-for-all with students determining their own curriculum from a range of options, with only placements remaining as compulsory. Those programmes which adopted systems theory were little different. It seemed that the main attraction of systems theory was that it permitted some opportunity for students to consider wider societal factors while continuing to preserve the primacy of the individual and family. This was how an American-social work educator put the case for systems theory:

> General systems theory may effectively meet the profession's current need for conceptual tools that activate an understanding of the relational determinants of behaviour in the person in the situation configuration. Systems theory is not in itself a body of knowledge; it is a way of thinking and of analysing that accommodates knowledge from many sciences. It offers a framework in which social interaction can be objectively understood without jeopardy to the work of individualisation.
>
> (Janchill, 1968: 77–8)

Even so, systems theory proved to be no replacement for psychoanalysis at the core of British social work's knowledge base. Unlike psychoanalysis, systems theory provided no energising vision or purpose, and its conservatism in failing to question the legitimacy and nature of the systems in which so many clients were locked was clearly transparent (Leonard, 1975: 78).

These were difficult years for the social-work academy. Cherished beliefs were being rejected by students from within the courses and outside in the agencies. Many social-work tutors had little experience of how to manage this new context of strife and conflict, and intellectually they were often humiliatingly exposed. Appeals to students that they were joining an honourable profession with roots in Christian compassion and charity (Younghusband, 1952: 717) carried little conviction with those who rejected traditional social-work histories which glorified heroines and heroes of charitable endeavour. New developments in social history inspired by the work of writers such as E.P. Thompson were exposing such accounts as little more than ideological dross and deeply misleading (Gettleman, 1974; G.S. Jones, 1971).

DANGEROUS THEORY

The social science disciplines which had previously been pillaged to provide support for traditional social-work activity were now considered to be dangerous and threatening. One teacher of social workers in 1974, a sociologist as it happens, noted that sociology had become a difficult subject to teach to social workers as it so easily gave rise to 'confusion and despondency'. He continued: 'Such an accusation cannot be dismissed lightly. The dangers of undermining the professional commitments of novices in the field parallel those of putting a viper in the cradle of an infant' (Wilson, 1974: 9). This is extraordinary language in which to discuss a subject which had been a key contributory discipline for social-work education since its origins in the School of Sociology created in 1902 by the COS. But Wilson's concern was not so much with the previously valued functionalist sociology identified by Heraud and Leonard a decade earlier, but with the critical sociology which social-work lecturers such as Munday had more specifically identified:

> current theories in the sociology of deviance pose the greatest threat of all to social work students with their clear message that society creates deviants for its own ends and that social workers as part of the system of social control, are used to create and amplify deviance rather than improve the lot of the deviant. The

ideas of writers like Matza, Becker, Cicourel are intellectually
fascinating and persuasive but quite ominous for the social
workers.

(Munday 1972: 4)

This sociology, as with other critical currents in psychology and
social policy, was threatening to state social work not because it was
'intellectually fascinating' but because it suggested some very clear
possibilities for a social-work practice which identified the concerns
of the clients as the central focus of the activity. Not only did such
material tend to construct clients as victims of oppressive social
relations and inequalities in power and resources, but in the process
problematised the role of the state and its social workers. In so doing,
these social sciences challenged the profoundly anti-democratic and
unaccountable model of state welfare professionalism which had
flourished under social democracy. Under that schema professionals,
on account of their training and certification, were deemed to be
experts with legitimate authority to define problems and determine
interventions. The client/patient/pupil/ . . ., as non-specialists, with
neither certificate nor degree, were accorded few if any rights in
defining their needs or preferred strategies. Within the changing
social-work occupation of the early 1970s one of the key radical
impulses was anti-professionalism, with organisations of radical
social workers such as Case Con advocating alliances between
clients and social workers based on the pursuit of social justice.
According to one social-work writer at the time:

the most vocal and dynamic of the new recruits to social work are
anti-professionalism with its built-in paternalism and inequalities.
They do not see themselves as skilled experts dispensing therapy
to social misfits, but as community workers where the client is no
longer the sick person but the sick society.

(Rankin, 1970: 21)

Although some of the positions taken at that time by radical social
workers might now be considered as naïve and optimistic, nevertheless serious attention was given to developing alternative modes
of practice based on radical, feminist and progressive political
perspectives, informed and inspired by insights drawn from a range
of emergent critical texts which the traditional social-work academy
had great difficulty in countering. The social-work academy's long-
standing conditional and partial approach to theory, seeing it as a

resource to be plundered and pillaged to give the occupation legitimacy and authority, provided no means of defence. Moreover, its persistent anxiety from the time of the COS (Bosanquet, 1893; Gow, 1900; Bannatyne, 1902) that 'untamed' social theory was potentially a source of contamination, was being realised. Students were now posing a range of first-order questions about society, families, gender relations, sexuality and racism, and demonstrating an unwillingness to accept the prevailing social order and affecting low-level change in the lives of a few clients. In the face of these developments a vacuum emerged which was to be all too easily filled by the training and regulatory demands of the agencies. The social-work academy, unable to control these developments, was vulnerable to the demands of the employers and offered no notable resistance to a process of transformation which for the next twenty years was to witness the de-intellectualising of social-work education.

THE EMPLOYERS' TAKE-OVER

The upsurge of radicalism combined with the bureaucratisation of the Social Services Departments saw employers seriously question social-work courses and question the right of the academy to determine the curriculum and ethos of social-work education. In its Second Annual Report in 1975, CCETSW noted that employers were pressing the value of practical training and the necessity of social workers to 'understand the rules and regulations of the organisations for which they work, and to be efficient in carrying out practical tasks'. The Report continued:

> From this point of view there may be a tendency to undervalue the academic disciplines that the students are being taught or even to suspect that the education they receive makes them difficult employees more concerned to change the 'system' than to get on with the job. Clearly, social work education must balance these pressures.
>
> (CCETSW, 1975: 38–9)

The employers' attack on the academic content of courses arose precisely because of their concern that such education *at that time* was making for difficult employees. Their demand was for employees who would do as they were told, not for social workers who thought and acted as though they were autonomous professionals with obligations to enhance as they saw fit the well-being of clients.

In an earlier discussion paper on fieldwork training for students, one of CCETSW's immediate predecessors, the Council for Training in Social Work, also observed how the college-based components of social-work courses were creating tensions for agencies:

> students on most courses nowadays are familiar with new concepts about conflict and consensus, and some see conflict rather than co-operation as the only solution to certain social problems. This viewpoint may well be having a considerable and unexpected impact in some agencies. Teaching on organisations theory may also impose further strain on some fieldwork teachers, agencies and students. . . . All the foregoing pose fresh problems about students' obligations to adhere to agency policies.
>
> (CTSW, 1971: 19)

As the 1970s progressed, the clamour from agencies increased. The Certificate of Qualification in Social Work (CQSW) became a major target of agencies and their organisations. The focus of their critique was principally a variant on the old theme that students were being radicalised by their exposure to critical social science material, whether concerned with poverty, sexism, bureaucracy, profession-alism or deviancy. For some the social workers' strike towards the end of the decade was no more than the consequence of students coming off their CQSW courses 'armed with the little red books on the thoughts of Chairman Mao' (Coventry councillor, cited in *Social Work Today*, 27 Feb. 1979, p. ii). Needless to say, many of the criticisms were exaggerated, for there were very few CQSW courses, maybe one or two which openly embraced a progressive stance. The problem was that many courses, no matter how traditional, were no longer able to guarantee the appropriate regulation and control over the new recruits.

For many state agencies these developments were taken as evidence that CQSW courses were unreliable and that the social-work academy could not be entrusted with professional education. It was at this juncture that the academy's traditional leadership role within British social work, at least in the period since 1945, was taken over by agency representatives and managers. CCETSW became a site of engagement with successive Conservative adminis-trations committed to increasing the representation of business and employers and in ensuring that it became effective in regulating, determining and shaping the nature of social-work education in the interests of the major employers. As Brewster, a critical voice from within CCETSW, noted, the composition of the Council by 1990 had seen representation from higher education eclipsed by the 'new managers' (Brewster, 1992: 88). He also claimed that 'CCETSW is now becoming an almost perfectly designed vehicle for the 'Thatch-erite' enterprise' (1992: 91).

Even the most cursory examination of CCETSW's development over the past 20 years bears out Brewster's assessment. Contrast, for example, the following statements. In 1971, CTSW acknowledged that

> it is vitally important that students' educational experience should engage their enthusiasm for social reform and social action, and help them to understand better the range of social problems and the complexities of reform. They should be given the opportunities to express, examine and analyse their criticisms of the actions of social workers and social agencies.

(1971: 19)

By May 1976, CCETSW was condemning students and college staff who were not prepared to compromise their principles, and accusing students of wanting to escape

> into social comment and well informed criticisms of society, and of social service structure, of the value bases of social work and of the 'subjectivity' of social work intervention. Such an escape is sometimes aided by college teachers who are usually protected from situations where professional judgements have to be made and consequences faced – akin to not facing and evading the failing student which so many find difficult.

(CCETSW, 1976: 13)

THE INTELLECTUAL PURGE

From this time onwards, as I have detailed elsewhere (Jones 1989, 1993, 1994), CCETSW, under pressure from both employers and successive Conservative governments, has proceeded to rip out the social science disciplines from the curriculum and remove the control of the academy over professional courses. In doing so it played on the philistinism of the New Right and its fear of intellectuals and education. Universities are sneered at as being ivory towers far removed from the pressures of everyday life; theorisation is deemed as escape, or even a symptom of a cold and uncaring personality; what is demanded of state welfare workers is obedience and loyalty, not thought. Ministers responsible for state social work have attempted to demean theorisation as 'fashionable' and of having no place in social-work activity. In its place, they demand common sense, which, as Lousada has rightly noted, is 'a defence against not knowing . . . and the high priest of what Bion referred to as 'anti-thought', or as Jacoby wrote, "common sense is the half truths of a deceitful society"' (1993: 112). Consequently, subjects which were once in the core of the curriculum have been virtually stripped out or given so little space in the timetable that they are without influence. Training rather than education predominates. Under the current Diploma in Social Work regulations stipulated by CCETSW, social science teaching and inputs are only permitted where they are deemed to be directly relevant to the social-work task. Course units on the sociology of organisations and bureaucracies which were relatively common on many professional courses in the 1970s are no longer possible under the new arrangements. Since 1975, CCETSW has made it clear that the contribution of the social sciences to the social-work enterprise is both to be limited and controlled. Non-professionally qualified social science lecturers can no longer determine their curriculum when it comes to the teaching of social workers, and they have been prevented since 1975 as acting as tutors for students on placements. On many programmes such social science lecturers have disappeared altogether.

That there has been relatively little opposition to this process from within the social-work academy requires some explanation. In part it is to be found in the kind of comments made by Munday and Wilson noted above, who represent a long tradition within the social-work academy. As the social sciences evolved in the twentieth century and moved away from their foundations as disciplines primarily concerned with seeking conservative solutions to the social upheavals and distress consequent upon capitalist development, so social work has found them to be more uncomfortable bedfellows. There is now prevailing within British social-work education a view epitomised by CCETSW, that social science knowledge is *not relevant* to social workers. This is probably correct if one defines social work only in terms of being a specific activity sanctioned by the state. It is clearly not true if one believes that social work is an activity concerned with enhancing human and social welfare.

The lack of opposition from students and front-line workers also needs to be considered. There is no simple explanation and, as we have argued elsewhere (Jones and Novak, 1993), a multiplicity of factors have contributed to a general state of demoralisation and exhaustion within the social-work occupation which has taken its toll in terms of undermining resistance and activism. It is not a wholly gloomy picture as evidenced by the initiatives taken by social workers, students and community organisations with regard to anti-racism, which was very much a campaign from below and for a tantalisingly brief moment in the late 1980s and early 1990s was able to press CCETSW to incorporate anti-racist commitments into the new regulations for the Dip SW. This was something of an exception, for over the past 15 years, the remorseless attacks on social workers in the tabloid media (encouraged by Conservative governments), especially around the physical and sexual abuse of children and the murders and deaths of youngsters in 'the care' or under the supervision of social workers, has induced a climate of caution in social work. Students and fieldworkers as well as their agency managers, albeit for different reasons, have tended to adopt defensive procedures in order to protect themselves from potential tabloid persecution. An occupation that now relies on compliance to a series of regulations and procedures to determine and direct much of its work understandably is drawn to training and competencies rather than education, research and understanding.

POSSIBILITIES

There are, nevertheless, countless social workers in Britain and elsewhere whose practice has been decisively informed by knowledge and understanding derived from the social sciences, and particularly from what might be described as its radical and critical currents. Feminist scholarship, for example, has provided many new critical insights into the processes and consequences of patriarchy, which in turn have influenced the practice of many social workers working with women and children who are no longer prepared to pathologise women or lone mothers, and who challenge long-standing notions about a 'woman's (subordinate) place'. Likewise, the texts which have researched racism and the struggles and oppressions of black people in British society have provided social workers committed to anti-racism with incontrovertible evidence of the endemic nature of racism in this society, whatever Geoffrey Greenwood, the current Chair of CCETSW, might otherwise claim. Committed anti-racist social workers know that he is wrong not solely on the basis of some competing value-orientation but on the basis of research and knowledge. As with sexism and other persistent forms of oppression and discrimination, including homophobia, disablism and ageism, research and scholarship has provided powerful new insights which can and do influence social-work practice. Those social workers who have determinedly resisted the anti-intellectual traditions of social work, who have refused to accept that theory is irrelevant to practice, have in unheralded fashion created methods and practice strategies which at their very least do not pathologise their clients and which swim against the tide of demonisation which is so prevalent in Britain today.

Such activities and developments are being increasingly squeezed to the very margins of social work in Britain. Precisely because they offer insights and methods of emancipatory practice which challenge the legitimacy of prevailing social arrangements and deepening inequalities, there has been an intellectual purging of the social-work curriculum. The recent convulsions within CCETSW over the requirements concerning anti-racism which have been dropped with inelegant haste because of government disapproval is but one example of such purging. Likewise the recent review of the Dip SW demanded by the government before the first cohort of entrants had completed, is indicative not only of social work's feeble position – what other so called profession would have tolerated such interference? – but also the government's persistence in seeking to stamp its authority over the future development of social-work education. The review, as it happens, does not propose many changes; nevertheless, it was an opportunity for the occupation to demand a three-year period for the Dip SW as against the current two years. No such demands were made. The national curriculum for social work as set out by CCETSW is simply ridiculous. It positively endorses 'anti-thinking' as there is no other way of managing the vastness of the curriculum.

END NOTE

As state personal social service agencies have been compelled to adhere to the New Right's social policy agenda of managing the exclusion of marginal and surplus (to labour market requirements) populations of reducing their social costs and therefore rights, so professional social-work courses have been brought under closer control and scrutiny. Colleges and social-work academics are no longer entrusted with social-work education. It is not that they were radical or oppositional, for as noted above they have in the main operated with the intention of securing the loyalty of future social workers and constructed and delivered curricula intent upon the immunisation of social workers from the ever-present danger of radical contamination or demoralisation. They lost control because they could no longer guarantee such immunisation.

The creation of the CSS in 1975 through to the latest review of the Diploma in Social Work in 1994/95 is a story of British social-work education accommodating the demands of an increasingly authoritarian state in which the role and nature of social work are being transformed. It is a process which has and is continuing to involve the demonisation of major elements of social work's client populations in order to legitimate the policy imperatives of increased surveillance and fewer resources. In this context, Social Services Departments need a social-work service capable of being managed, not one that has illusions of autonomous or professional practice. Clients and their needs cannot, even at the level of rhetoric, be the pivotal focus of the activity. Instead, the foremost duty of the state social worker is loyalty and obedience to the agency. From the mid-1970s this has been reinforced by the introduction and subsequent modification of contracts of employment, most of which now contain clear disciplinary consequences for social workers who speak to the press or reporters, infringe the law however trivially, or refuse to accept the instructions of managers.

The same concerns have propelled agency managers into the universities and colleges where they now 'share' responsibility with tutors and lecturers for the organisation and delivery of the curric-ulum. Their demands for social workers who come off courses ready to do the job asked of them without question have led to the narrow focus on training and competencies. As one Director of a Social Services Department in a northern city declared when discussing the development of a Dip SW programme, 'I want doers not thinkers.' In the current context, thinkers are dangerous. That is precisely why, in any reconceptualisation and reconstruction of British social work as an activity that is committed to social justice and human welfare, that might conceivably have a part to play in more enlightened future, we must break with a century of tradition in social-work education and demand the right to debate, to think, to study and research.

In pressing these claims, we should clearly distinguish our demand for education from that made for most of the twentieth century where education for social workers has been driven by concerns to inculcate conservative and elitist perspectives. The domain of social work is compelling, important and contested. It demands and requires integrity, enquiry, debate and research. Above all, it demands new partnerships in the formation of its knowledge base and curricula which involve the users of services and those social constituencies which have hitherto been considered as not counting. This is where the agenda for a new social-work education must be set if we are serious about empowerment and anti-oppressive practice. It can't be done with or under managers of state agencies, or for that matter with CCETSW, nor should it be left to the academics. It is a project of some urgency.

References

Abbott, P. and Wallace, C. (1992) *The Family and the New Right*, London: Pluto Press.

Advisory Council on the Penal System (1970) *Non-Custodial and Semi-Custodial Penalties* (Wootton Report), London: HMSO.

—— (1974) *Young Adult Offenders* (Younger Report), London: HMSO.

Aglietta, M. (1979) *A Theory of Capitalist Regulation*, London: Verso.

Alaszewski, A. and Manthorpe, J. (1991) 'Literature Review: Measuring and Managing Risk in Social Welfare', *British Journal of Social Work*, 21 (3): 277–90.

Aldridge, M. (1994) *Making Social Work News*, London: Routledge.

Allan, G. (1991) 'Social Work, Community Care and Informal Networks', in M. Davies (ed.), *The Sociology of Social Work*, London: Routledge, pp. 106–22.

Anderson, P. (1968) 'Components of the National Culture', *New Left Review*, 50: 3–57.

Anon. (1968) 'Sociology and Social Work', *Child Care News*, 77: 11–12.

Association of Chief Officers of Probation (ACOP) (1994) *Guidance on the Management of Risk and Public Protection*, London: Association of Chief Officers of Probation.

Audit Commission (1989) *The Probation Service: Promoting Value for Money*, London: HMSO.

—— (1991) *Going Straight: Developing Good Practice in Probation*, Occasional Paper No. 16, London: HMSO.

—— (1992) *The Community Revolution: the Personal Social Services and Community Care*, London: HMSO.

—— (1994) *Seen but Not Heard: Co-ordinating Child Health and Social Services for Children in Need*, London: HMSO.

Avineri, S. and de-Shalit, A. (eds) (1992) *Communitarianism and Individualism*, Oxford: Oxford University Press.

Aziz, R. (1992) 'Feminism and the Challenge of Racism: Deviance or Difference?', in H. Crowley and S. Himmelweit (eds), *Knowing Women*, Cambridge: Polity Press.

Baher, E., Hyman, C., Jones, C., Jones, R., Kerr, A. and Mitchell, R. (1976) *At Risk: an Account of the Work of the Battered Child Research Department*, London: Routledge & Kegan Paul.

Bailey, R. and Brake, M. (eds) (1975) *Radical Social Work*, London: Edward Arnold.

Baldock, J. (1994) 'The Personal Social Services: the Politics of Care', in V. George and F. Miller (eds) *Social Policy towards 2000: Squaring the Welfare Circle*, London: Routledge.

Bamford, T. (1990) *The Future of Social Work*, London: Macmillan.

Bannatyne, K. V. (1902) 'The Place and Training of Volunteers in Charitable Work', *Charity Organisation Review* (June): 332–47.

Barrett, M. (1987) 'The Concept of Difference', *Feminist Review*, 26: 29–41.

—— (1991) *The Politics of Truth: From Marx to Foucault*, Cambridge: Polity Press.

—— (1992) 'Words and Things: Materialism and Method in Contemporary Feminist Analysis', in M. Barrett and A. Phillips (eds) *Destabilizing Theory: Contemporary Feminist Debates*, Cambridge: Polity Press

Barrett, M. and Phillips, A. (eds) (1992) *Destabilizing Theory: Contemporary Feminist Debates*, Cambridge: Polity Press.

Barthes, R. (1977) 'The Death of the Author', in *Image-Music-Test*, trans. S. Heath, London: Fontana Books.

Baudrillard, J. (1975) *The Mirror of Production*, trans. M. Poster, St Louis, MO: Telos Press.

—— (1992) *The Mirror of Production*, trans. M. Poster, St Louis, MO: Telos Press.

Bauman, Z. (1987) *Legislators and Interpreters: On Modernity, Postmodernity and Intellectuals*, Cambridge: Polity Press.

—— (1991) *Modernity and Ambivalence*, Cambridge: Polity Press.

—— (1992) *Intimations of Postmodernity*, London: Routledge.

Beazley, M. (1994) 'Measuring Service Quality', in N. Malin (ed.) *Implementing Community Care*, Milton Keynes: Open University Press, pp. 122–37.

Beck, U. (1992a) *Risk Society: Towards a New Modernity*, London: Sage.

—— (1992b) 'From Industrial Society to Risk Society: Questions of Survival, Social Structure and Ecological Enlightenment', *Theory, Culture and Society*, 9 (1): 97–123.

Becker, S. and Silburn, R. (1990) *The New Poor Clients*, London: Community Care/Benefits Research Unit.

Bell, D. (1993) *Communitarianism and its Critics*, Oxford: Clarendon Press.

Benney, M. (1936) *Low Company: Describing the Evolution of a Burglar*, London: Peter Davies.

—— (1948) *Good Delivery*, London: Longmans, Green & Co.

Berthoud, R. (1990) *The Social Fund – Is It Working?* London: Policy Studies Institute.

Black, J., Bowl, R., Burns, D., Critcher, C., Grant, G. and Stockford, D. (1983) *Social Work in Context*, London: Tavistock.

Bochel, D. (1976) *Probation and After-care: Its Development in England and Wales*, Edinburgh: Scottish Academic Press.

Booth, W. (1961) *The Rhetoric of Fiction*, Chicago: University of Chicago Press.

Bosanquet, B. (1893) *The Civilisation of Christendom*, London: Swan Sonnenschein.

—— (1916) 'The Philosophy of Casework', *Charity Organisation Review*, 39: 117–38.

Bottoms, A. E. (1977) 'Reflections on the Renaissance of Dangerousness', *Howard Journal of Penology and Crime Prevention*, 16 (2): 70–96.

Bottoms, A. and Brownsword, R. (1983) 'Dangerousness and Rights', in J. W. Hinton, (ed.), *Dangerousness: Problems of Assessment and Prediction*, London: Allen & Unwin.

Boyne, R. and Rattansi, A. (eds) (1990) *Postmodernism and Society*, London: Macmillan.

Brah, A. (1992) 'Difference, Diversity and Differentiation', in J. Donald and A. Rattansi (eds), *Race, Culture and Society*, London: Sage.

—— (1993) 'Reframing Europe: Engendered Racisms, Ethnicities and Nationalisms in Contemporary Western Europe', in *Feminist Review*, 45: 9–28.

Brearley, C. P. (1982) *Risk and Social Work*, London: Routledge & Kegan Paul.

Brearley, C. P. with Hall, M., Jeffreys, P., Jennings, R. and Pritchard, S. (1982) *Risk and Ageing*, London: Routledge & Kegan Paul.

Brewster, R. (1992) 'The New Class? Managerialism and Social Work Education and Training', *Issues in Social Work Education*, 11 (2): 81–93.

Britton, C. (1954) 'Child Care', in C Morris (ed.), *Social Casework in Great Britain*, London: Faber.

Bryman, A. (1993) 'The Nature of Organisation Structure: Constraint and Choice', in D. Morgan and L. Stanley (eds), *Debates in Sociology*, Manchester: Manchester University Press.

Burrows, R. and Loader, B. (eds) (1994) *Towards a Post-Fordist Welfare State?* London: Routledge.

Bury, M. (1994) *Ageing and Sociological Theory: a Critique*, paper presented at Ageing and Gender Conference, University of Surrey (July).

Butrym, Z. (1976) *The Nature of Social Work*, London: Macmillan.

Bytheway, B. (1994) 'Ageism and the Conceptualisation of Age', paper presented at British Society of Gerontology Conference (Sept.), London.

Caldock, K. (1993) 'A Preliminary Study of Changes in Assessment: Examining the Relationship between Recent Policy and Practitioners' Knowledge, Opinions and Practice', *Health and Social Care in the Community*, 1 (3): 139–46.

Caldock, K. and Nolan, M. (1994) 'Assessment and Community Care: Are the Reforms Working?', *Generations Review*, 4 (4): 2–7.

Callinicos, A. (1989) *Against Postmodernism: a Marxist Critique*, Cambridge: Polity Press.

—— (1990) 'Reactionary Postmodernism', in R. Boyne and A. Rattansi (eds), *Postmodernism and Society*, Basingstoke: Hutchinson.

Campbell, J. C. (1995) *Assessing Dangerousness: Violence by Sexual Offenders, Batterers, and Child Abusers*, London: Sage.

Carby, H. (1982) 'White Woman Listen! Black Feminism and the Boundaries of Sisterhood', in *The Empire Strikes Back*, London: Hutchinson.

CCETSW (1975) *Second Annual Report*, London, CCETSW.

—— (1976) *Guidelines to Social Work Training Rules 1975*, London: CCETSW.

—— (1989) *Requirements and Regulations for the Diploma in Social Work*, Paper 30, London: CCETSW.

—— (1991) *Rules and Requirements for the Diploma in Social Work*, Paper 30 (2nd edn), London: CCETSW.

—— (1994a) *UK Consultations on the 'Firm Draft' Requirements for the Revised Dipsw*, London: CCETSW.

—— (1994b) *Annual Report 1992–3*, London: CCETSW.

Charlesworth, J., Clarke, J. and Cochrane, A. (1994a) 'Managing Local Mixed Economies of Care', paper to Institute of British Geographers Conference (Jan.), Nottingham.

—— (1994b) 'Tangled Webs? Managing Local Mixed Economies of Care', paper to Employment Research Unit (Sept.), Cardiff.

Cheetham, J. (1993) 'Social Work and Community Care in the 1990s: Pitfalls and Potential', in R. Page and J. Baldock (eds), *Social Policy Review*, 5, Canterbury: Social Policy Association, pp. 155–76.

Clarke, J. (1991) *New Times and Old Enemies: Essays on Cultural Studies and America*, London: HarperCollins.

—— (1993a) *A Crisis in Care? Challenges to Social Work*, London: Sage.

—— (1993b) 'The Comfort of Strangers: Social Work in Context', in J. Clarke (ed.), *A Crisis in Care*, London: Sage.

—— (1994) 'Capturing the Customer: Consumerism and Social Welfare', paper to ESRC Seminar, 'Conceptualising Consumption Issues' (Dec.), Lancaster.

—— (forthcoming) 'Towards a Post-Fordist Welfare State', *Local Government Studies*.

Clarke, J., Cochrane, A. and McLaughlin, E. (eds) (1994) *Managing Social Policy*, London: Sage.

Clarke, J. and Critcher, C. (1984) *The Devil Makes Work: Leisure in Capitalist Britain*, Basingstoke: Macmillan.

Clarke, J. and Newman, J. (1993a) 'The Right to Manage: a Second Managerial Revolution?', *Cultural Studies*, 7 (3): 427–41.

—— (1993b) 'Managing to Survive? Dilemmas of Changing Organisational Forms in the Public Sector', in N. Deakin and R. Page (eds), *The Costs of Welfare*, Aldershot: Avebury.

—— (forthcoming) 'Managers, Markets and Mixed Economies', in F. Williams (ed.), *Social Policy: a Critical Reader*, Cambridge: Polity Press.

Clement Brown, S. (1945) 'Training for Social Work', *Social Work* (Oct.), 181–9.

Cochrane, A. (1989) 'Restructuring the State: the Case of Local Government', in A. Cochrane and J. Anderson (eds), *Politics in Transition*, London: Sage.

—— (1993a) 'Poverty', in R. Dallas and E. McLaughlin (eds), *Social Problems and the Family*, London: Sage.

—— (1993b) *Whatever Happened to Local Government?* Buckingham: Open University Press.

Cochrane, A. and Clarke, J. (eds) (1993) *Comparing Welfare States*, London: Sage.

Cohen, S. (1985) *Visions of Social Control: Crime, Punishment and Classification*, Cambridge: Polity Press.

—— (1994) 'Social Control and the Politics of Reconstruction', in D. Nelken (ed.), *The Futures of Criminology*, London: Sage.

Connor, S. (1989) *Postmodernist Culture: an Introduction to Theories of the Contemporary*, Oxford: Basil Blackwell.

Conrad, C. (1992) 'Old Age in the Modern and Postmodern Western World', in T. Cole, D. Van Tassel and R. Kastenbaum (eds), *Handbook of the Humanities and Ageing*, Springer Publishing Co. pp. 62–95.

Cooks, R. (1958) *Keep Them Out of Prison*, London: Jarrolds.

Cooper, C. and Davidson, M. (1982) *High Pressure – Working Lives of Women Managers*, London: Fontana.

Corrigan, P. and Leonard, P. (1978) *Social Work Practice under Capitalism: a Marxist Approach*, London: Macmillan.

Crook, S., Pakulski, J. and Waters, M. (1992) *Postmodernization: Change in Advanced Society*, London: Sage.

Crossman, R. (1969) Personal communication.

—— (1977) *The Diaries of a Cabinet Minister*, vol. III, London: Hamilton & Cage.

CTSW (1971) 'The Teaching of Fieldwork', *Discussion Paper No. 4*, London: CTSW.

Curtis Committee (1946) *Report of the Care of Children Committee*, London: HMSO.

Cutler, T. and Waine, B. (1994) *Managing the Welfare State: the Politics of Public Sector Management*, Oxford: Berg.

Dark, S. (1939) *Inasmuch . . . Christianity in the Police Courts*, London: Student Christian Movement Press.

Davies, M. (1985) *The Essential Social Worker*, (2nd edn), Aldershot: Gower.

—— (1991) 'Sociology and Social Work: a Misunderstood Relationship', in M. Davies (ed.) *The Sociology of Social Work*, London: Routledge.

Deed, D. (1953) 'The General Principles of Social Casework', *The Almoner*, 6 (6): 305–13.

Denman, G. and Thorpe, D. (1993) *Family Participation and Patterns of Intervention in Child Protection in Gwent*, Department of Applied Social Science, Lancaster University.

DHSS (1970) *The Battered Baby*, MO2/70.

—— (1972) *Battered Babies*, LASSL 26/72.

—— (1974) *Non-Accidental Injury to Children*, LASSL (74) (13).

—— (1976) *Non-Accidental Injury to Children: the Police and Case Conferences*, LASSC (76) (26).

—— (1982) *Child Abuse: a Study of Inquiry Reports 1973–1981*, London: HMSO.

—— (1985a) *Review of Child Care Law: Report to Ministers of an Interdepartmental Working Party*, London: HMSO.

—— (1985b) *Social Work Decisions in Child Care: Recent Research Findings and their Implications*, London: HMSO.

Dillon, C. (1969) 'The Professional Name Game', *Social Carework*, 50, (June).

Dingwall, R. (1989) 'Some Problems about Predicting Child Abuse and Neglect' in O. Stevenson, (ed.) *Child Abuse: Public Policy and Professional Practice*, Hemel Hempstead: Harvester Wheatsheaf.

Ditch, J. (1993) 'Next Steps: the Restructuring of Social Security', in N. Deakin and R. Page (eds), *The Costs of Welfare*, Aldershot: Avebury.

Docherty, T. (1987) *On Modern Authority: the Theory and Condition of Writing: 1500 to the Present Day*, Brighton: Harvester Press.

DoH (1988) *Protecting Children: a Guide for Social Workers Undertaking a Comprehensive Assessment*, London: HMSO.

—— (1989) *Caring for People: Community Care in the Next Decade and Beyond*, London: HMSO.

—— (1991a) *Working Together under the Children Act 1989*, London: HMSO.

—— (1991b) *Child Abuse: a Study of Inquiry Reports 1980–89*, London: HMSO.

—— (1994) *Children Act Report 1993*, London: HMSO.

Dominelli, L. (1991) 'What's in a Name? A Comment on 'Puritans and Paradigms'', *Social Sciences and Social Work Review*, 2 (3): 231–5.

Donzelot, J. (1979) *The Policing of Families*, London: Hutchinson.

—— (1988) 'The Promotion of the Social', *Economy and Society*, 17 (3): 395–427.

Douglas, M. (1986) *Risk Acceptability according to the Social Sciences*, London: Routledge & Kegan Paul.

—— (1992) *Risk and Blame: Essays in Cultural Theory*, London: Routledge.

Du Gay, P. (forthcoming) 'Organising Identity: Entrepreneurial Governance and Public Sector Management', in S. Hall and P. du Gay (eds), *Questions of Cultural Identity*, London: Sage.

Eco, U. (1979) *The Role of the Reader: Explorations in the Semiotics of Texts*, Bloomington: Indiana University Press.

Eley, R. (1987) 'Women at the Top', *Insight*, 2 (12): 12–14.

Evandrou, M., Falkingham, J. and Glennerster, H. (1990) 'The Personal Social Services: Everyone's Poor Relation but Nobody's Baby', in J. Hilk (ed.), *The State of Welfare: the Welfare State in Britain since 1974*, Oxford: Clarendon Press.

Featherstone, M. and Hepworth, M. (1989) 'Ageing and Old Age: Reflections on the Postmodern Life Course', in B. Bytheway, T. Keil, P. Allott and A. Bryman (eds), *Becoming and Being Old: Sociological Approaches to Later Life*, London: Sage, pp. 143–57.

—— (1994) 'Images of Ageing', in J. Bond, P. Coleman and S. Peace (eds), *Ageing in Society*, London: Sage, pp. 304–32.

Feeley, M. and Simon, J. (1994) 'Actuarial Justice: the Emerging New Criminal Law', in D. Nelkin (ed.), *The Future of Criminology*, London: Sage.

Fido, J. (1977) 'The Charity Organisation Society and Social Casework in London 1969–1900', in A. P. Donajgrodski (ed.), *Social Control in Nineteenth Century Britain*, London: Croom Helm.

Fielding, N. (1984) *Probation Practice: Client Support under Social Control*, Aldershot: Gower.

Finch, J. and Wallis, L. (1994) 'Inheritance, Care Bargains and Elderly People's Relationships with their Children', in D. Challis, B. Davies and

K. Traske (eds), *Community Care: New Agendas and Challenges from the UK and Overseas*, Aldershot: Gower, pp. 110–20.

Fischer, J. (1976) *The Effectiveness of Social Casework*, Illinois: Charles C. Thomas.

Flin, R. and Tarrant, M. (1989) 'Children in the Witness Box' *Social Work Today*, 21 (Feb.): 18–19.

Floud, J. and Young, W. (1981) *Dangerousness and Criminal Justice*, London: Heinemann.

Flynn, N. (1994) 'Control, Commitment and Contracts', in J. Clarke, A. Cochrane and E. McLaughlin (eds), *Managing Social Policy*, London: Sage.

Foster, J. (1991) 'The Under-representation of Women in Social Services Management', unpublished PhD thesis, University of Lancaster.

Foucault, M. (1977) *Discipline and Punish: the Birth of the Prison*, trans. A. Sheridan, Harmondsworth: Allen Lane.

—— (1981) *The History of Sexuality*, vol. I: *An Introduction*, trans. R. Hurley, Harmondsworth: Penguin Books.

Franklin, B. (ed.) (1986) *The Rights of Children*, London: Basil Blackwell.

—— (1995) *The Handbook of Children's Rights: Essay in Comparative Policy and Practice*, London: Routledge.

Franklin, R. and Parton, N. (eds) (1991) *Social Work, the Media and Public Relations*, London: Routledge.

Freeman, M. D. A. (1983) *The Rights and Wrongs of Children*, London: Francis Pinter.

—— (1987–88) 'Taking Children's Rights Seriously', *Children and Society*, 1 (4) (Winter): 299–319.

Gadamer, H-G. (1975) *Truth and Method*, London: Sheed & Ward.

Garland, D. (1985) *Punishment and Welfare: a History of Penal Strategies*, Aldershot: Gower.

Geach, H. and Szwed, E. (eds) (1983) *Providing Civil Justice for Children*, London: Arnold.

Genette, G. (1980) *Narrative Discourse*, trans. J. Lewin, Oxford: Basil Blackwell.

Gergen, K. (1991) *The Saturated Self: Dilemmas of Identity in Contemporary Life*, New York: Basic Books.

Gettleman, M. E. (1974) 'The Whig Interpretation of Social Welfare History', *Smith College Studies in Social Work*, xliv (3): 149–57.

Gibbons, J., Conroy, S. and Bell, C. (1993) *Operation of Child Protection Registers*, report to Department of Health, Norwich: Social Work Development Unit, University of East Anglia.

Giddens, A. (1990) *The Consequences of Modernity*, Cambridge: Polity Press.

—— (1991) *Modernity and Self-Identity: Self and Society in the Late Modern Age*, Cambridge: Polity Press.

Gilbert, B. (1966) *The Evolution of National Insurance in Great Britain*, London: Michael Joseph.

Giller, H., Gormley, C. and Williams, P. (1992) *The Effectiveness of Child Protection Procedures*, Manchester: Social Information Systems.

Goldberg, E. M. (1974) *Journal of Psychosomatic Research*, 18.

Goodman, A. and Webb, S. (1994) *For Richer, for Poorer: the Changing Distribution of Income in the United Kingdom*, 1961–91, London: Institute for Fiscal Studies.

Gordon, L. (1992) *Heroes of Their Own Lives*, London: Verso.

Gow, H. J. (1900) 'Methods of Training', *Charity Organisation Review*, 8 (44): 109–15.

Graham, H. (1992) 'Feminism and Social Work Education', *Issues in Social Work Education*, 11 (2): 48–64.

Gray, A. and Jenkins, B. (1993) 'Markets, Managers and the Public Service: the Changing of a Culture', in P. Taylor-Gooby and R. Lawson (eds), *Markets and Managers: New Issues in the Delivery of Welfare*, Buckingham: Open University Press.

Griffin, G., Hester, M., Rai, S. and Roseneil, S. (1994) *Stirring It: Challenges for Feminism*, London: Taylor & Francis.

Grünhut, M. (1948) *Penal Reform: a Comparative Study*, Oxford: Clarendon Press.

Gubrium, J. F. (1988) 'Incommunicable and Poetic Documentation in the Alzheimer's Disease Experience', *Semiotica*, 72: 235–53.

Hacking, I. (1975) *The Emergence of Probability: A Philosophical Study of Early Ideas about Probability, Induction and Statistical Inferences*, Cambridge: Cambridge University Press.

Hall, P. (1976) *Reforming the Welfare*, London: Heinemann.

Hallett, C. and Birchall, E. (1992) *Coordination and Child Protection: a Review of the Literature*, London: HMSO.

Halmos, P. (1965) *The Faith of the Counsellors*, London: Constable.

Harden, I. (1992) *The Contracting State*, Basingstoke: Macmillan.

Harding, T. (1992) 'Questions on the Social Services Agenda', in T. Harding (ed.), *Who Owns Welfare? Questions on the Social Services Agenda*, Social Services Policy Forum Paper II, London: National Institute for Social Work.

Harris, R. (1990) 'A Matter of Balance: Power and Resistance in Child Protection Policy', *Journal of Social Welfare Law*, 5: 332–40.

—— (1992) *Crime, Criminal Justice and the Probation Service*, London: Routledge.

—— (1994) 'Continuity and Change: Probation and Politics in Contemporary Britain', *International Journal of Offender Therapy and Comparative Criminology*, 38: 33–45.

—— (1995) 'Probation Round the World: Origins and Development', in K. Hamai, R. Ville, R. Harris, M. House and U. Zvekic (eds), *Probation Round the World: a Comparative Study*, London: Routledge.

Harris, R. and Timms, N. (1993) *Secure Accommodation and Child Care: Between Hospital and Prison or Thereabouts*, London: Routledge.

Harris, R. and Webb, D. (1987) *Welfare, Power and Juvenile Justice: the Social Control of Delinquent Youth*, London: Tavistock Publications.

Harrison, S. and Pollitt, C. (1994) *Controlling Health Professionals: the Future of Work and Organization in the National Health Service*, Buckingham: Open University Press.

Harvey, D. (1989) *The Condition of Postmodernity: an Enquiry into the Origins of Cultural Change*, Oxford: Blackwell.

Haxby, D. (1978) *Probation: a Changing Service*, London: Constable.

Health Committee Second Report (1991) *Public Expenditure on Personal Social Services and Child Protection Services*, vol. 1, *Report together with the Proceedings of the Committee*, London: HMSO.

Heller, A. and Feher, K. (1988) *The Postmodern Political Condition*, Cambridge: Polity Press.

Henkel, M. (1991a) *Government, Evaluation and Change*, London: Jessica Kingsley.

—— (1991b) 'The New "Evaluative State"', *Public Administration*, 69: 121–36.

Henriques, B. (1950) *Indiscretions of a Magistrate; Thoughts on the Work of the Juvenile Court*, London: Harrap.

Heraud, B. (1967) 'Teaching of Sociology in Professional Social Work Courses', unpublished paper given to the Sociology Teachers Section of the British Sociological Association.

Hill-Collins, P. (1991) *Black Feminist Theory: Knowledge, Consciousness and the Politics of Employment*, London: Routledge.

Hills, J. (ed.) (1990) *The State of Welfare: the Welfare State in Britain since 1974*, London, Oxford University Press.

Hirst, P. (1981) 'The Genesis of the Social', *Politics and Power*, 3: 67–82.

Hobson, J. A. (1896) 'The Social Philosophy of Charity Organisation', *Contemporary Review*, 70: 710–27.

Hoggett, P. (1994) 'The Politics of the Modernisation of the UK Welfare State', in R. Burrows and B. Loader (eds), *Towards a Post-Fordist Welfare State?* London: Routledge.

Holmes, T. (1900) *Pictures and Problems from London Police Courts*, London: Edward Arnold.

Home Office (1972) *Report on the Work of the Probation and After-care Department 1969 to 1971*, Cmnd 5158, London: HMSO.

—— (1976) *Report on the Work of the Probation and After-care Department 1972–1975*, Cmnd 6590, London: HMSO.

—— (1984) *Probation Service in England and Wales: Statement of National Objectives and Priorities*, London: Home Office.

—— (1987) *Efficiency Scrutiny of Her Majesty's Probation Inspectorate* (Grimsey Report), London: Home Office.

Home Office in conjunction with the Department of Health (1992) *Memorandum of Good Practice on Video Recording with Child Witnesses for Criminal Proceedings*, London: HMSO.

Home Office, Department of Health, Department of Education and Science and Welsh Office (1991) *Working Together Under the Children Act 1989: a Guide to Arrangements for Inter-agency Co-operation for the Protection of Children from Abuse*, London: HMSO.

Hopkins, J. (1969) Personal communication with the Secretary of State.

Howe, A. (1994) *Punish and Critique: Towards a Feminist Analysis of Penality*, London: Routledge.

Howe, D. (1986) *Social Workers and their Practice in Welfare Bureaucracies*, Aldershot: Gower.

—— (1991) 'The Family and the Therapist: Towards a Sociology of Social

Work Method', in M. Davies (ed.), *The Sociology of Social Work*, London: Routledge, pp. 146–62.

—— (1992) 'Child Abuse and the Bureaucratization of Social Work', *Sociological Review*, 40 (3): 491–508.

—— (1994) 'Modernity, Postmodernity and Social Work', *British Journal of Social Work*, 24 (5): 513–32.

—— (1995) *Attachment Theory for Social Work Practice*, Basingstoke: Macmillan.

Howitt, D. C. (1992) *Child Abuse Errors: When Good Intentions Go Wrong*, London: Harvester Wheatsheaf.

Hudson, A. (1992) 'The Child Sexual Abuse Industry and Gender Relations in Social Work', in M. Langan and L. Day (eds), *Women, Oppression and Social Work*, London: Routledge.

Hudson, B. (1994) *Making Sense of Markets in Health and Social Care*, Sunderland: Business Education Publishers.

Hudson, R. (1988) 'Labour Markets and New Forms of Work in 'Old' Industrial Regions', in D. Massey and J. Allen (eds), *Uneven Development: Cities and Regions in Transition*, London: Hodder & Stoughton.

Hughes, B. (1993) 'A Model for the Comprehensive Assessment of Older People and their Carers', *British Journal of Social Work*, 23 (4): 345–65.

Hughes, E. (1951/71) *The Sociological Eye*, Chicago: Aldine-Atherton.

Hugman, R. (1994a) *Ageing and the Care of Older People in Europe*, London: Macmillan.

—— (1994b) 'Social Work and Case Management in the UK: Models of Professionalism and Older People', in *Ageing and Society*, 14 (2): 237–54.

Ingleby, D. (1985) 'Professionals as Socialisers: the "Psy" Complex', in A. Scully and S. Spitzer (eds), *Research in Law, Deviance and Social Control*, 7, New York: Jai Press.

Irvine, E. E. (1954) 'Research into Problem Families', *British Journal of Psychiatric Social Work*, 9, (Spring).

—— (1956) 'Some Implications of Freudian Theory for Casework', *The Almoner*, 9 (2): 39–44.

Jack, R. (1992) 'Case Management: Social Services Welfare or Trade Fare?' *Generations Review*, 2(1).

Jameson, F. (1991) *Postmodernism or the Cultural Logic of Late Capitalism*, London: Verso.

Janchill, M. P. (1968) 'Systems Concepts in Casework Theory and Practice', *Social Casework*, 50 (2): 74–82.

Jarvis, F. (1972) *Advise, Assist and Befriend: a History of the Probation and After-care Service*, London: Home Office.

Jessop, B. (1994) 'The Transition to Post-Fordism and the Schumpeteman Workfare State', in R. Burrows and B. Loader (eds), *Towards a Post-Fordist Welfare State?* London: Routledge.

Jones, C. (1978) 'An Analysis of the Development of Social Work Education and Social Work 1869–1977: The Making of Citizens and Super-citizens', unpublished PhD thesis, University of Durham.

—— (1983) *State Social Work and the Working Class*, London: Macmillan.

—— (1989) 'The End of the Road? Issues in Social Work Education', in P.

Carter, T. Jeffs and M. Smith (eds), *Social Work and Social Welfare Yearbook*, 1, Milton Keynes: Open University Press.

—— (1993) 'Distortion and Demonisation: the Right and Anti-racist Social Work Education', *Social Work Education*, 12 (12): 9–16.

—— (1994) 'Dangerous Times for British Social Work Education', unpublished paper given to the 27th Congress of the International Association of Social Work, Amsterdam (July).

Jones, C. and Novak, T. (1993) 'Social Work Today', *British Journal of Social Work*, 23 (2): 195–212.

Jones, G. S. (1971) *Outcast London*, Oxford: Clarendon Press.

Jordan, B., Redley, M. and Jones, S. (1994) *Putting the Family First: Identities, Decisions, Citizenship*, London: UCL Press.

Kelly, A. (1991) 'The 'New' Managerialism in Social Services', in P. Carter, T. Jeffs and M. Smith (eds), *Social Work and Social Welfare Yearbook*, 3, Buckingham: Open University Press.

Kempe, C. H., Silverman, F. N., Steele, B. F., Droegemueller, W. and Silver, H. K. (1962) 'The Battered Child Syndrome', *Journal of the American Medical Association*, 181: 17–24.

Kendall, K. (1972) 'Dream or Nightmare? The Future of Social Work Education', *Social Work Today*, 3 (16): 2–8.

King, J. (ed.) (1958) *The Probation Service*, London: Butterworth.

Krieger, J. (1987) 'Social Policy in the Age of Reagan and Thatcher', in R. Miliband *et al.* (eds), *Socialist Register 1987*, London: Merlin.

Langan, M. (1993a) 'The Rise and Fall of Social Work', in J. Clarke (ed.) *A Crisis in Care*, London: Sage.

—— (1993b) 'New Directions in Social Work', in J. Clarke (ed.), *A Crisis in Care*, London: Sage.

Langan, M. and Clarke, J. (1993) 'Restructuring Welfare: the British Welfare Regime in the 1980s', in A. Cochrane and J. Clarke (eds), *Comparing Welfare States*, London: Sage.

—— (1994) 'Managing in the Mixed Economy of Welfare', in J. Clarke, A. Cochrane and E. McLaughlin (eds), *Managing Social Policy*, London: Sage, pp. 73–92.

Lash, S. (1990) *Sociology of Postmodernism*, London: Routledge.

Laslett, P. (1994) 'The Third Age, the Fourth Age and the Future', in *Ageing and Society*, 14 (3): 436–47.

LeGrand, J. (1990) *Quasi-Markets and Social Policy*, School for Advanced Urban Studies, University of Bristol.

LeGrand, J. and Bartlett, W. (1993) *Quasi-Markets and Social Policy*, Basingstoke: Macmillan.

Leigh, J. (1992) 'The Child Support Act 1991: Its Relationship with the Children Act 1989', *Journal of Child Law*, 4: 177–80.

Le Mesurier, L (1931) *Boys in Court: a Study of Adolescent Crime and Its Treatment*, London: John Murray.

Leonard, P (1966) *Sociology and Social Work*, London: Routledge & Kegan Paul.

—— (1975) 'Poverty, Consciousness and Action', *Sheila Kay Memorial Lecture*, BASW.

Ling, T. (1994) 'Managing Social Security', in J. Clarke, A. Cochrane and E. McLaughlin (eds), *Managing Social Policy*, London: Sage.

Lister, R. (1993) 'Tracing the Contours of Women's Citizenship', *Policy and Politics*, 21 (1): 3–16.

Loader, B. and Burrows, R. (1994) 'Towards a Post-Fordist Welfare State: the Restructuring of Britain, Social Policy and the Future of Welfare', in R. Burrows and B. Loader (eds), *Towards a Post-Fordist Welfare State*, London: Routledge.

Locke, T. (1990) *New Approaches to Crime in the 1990s: Planning Responses to Crime*, London: Longman.

London Borough of Brent (1985) *A Child in Trust: Report of the Panel of Inquiry Investigating the Circumstances Surrounding the Death of Jasmine Beckford*, London: London Borough of Brent.

London Borough of Greenwich (1987) *A Child in Mind: Protection of Children in a Responsible Society, Report of the Commission of Inquiry into the Circumstances Surrounding the Death of Kimberley Carlile*, London: London Borough of Greenwich.

London Borough of Lambeth (1987) *Whose Child? The Report of the Panel Appointed to Inquire into the Death of Tyra Henry*, London: Borough of Lambeth.

Lorenz, W. (1994) *Social Work in a Changing Europe*, London: Routledge.

Lousada, J. (1993) 'Self-defence is No Offence', *Journal of Social Work Practice*, 7 (2): 103–13.

Lubove, R. (1966) 'Social Work and the Life of the Poor', *The Nation*, 23 May, pp. 609–11.

Luhman, N. (1993) *Risk: a Sociological Theory*, Berlin: Walter de Gryter.

McBeath, G. B. and Webb, S. A. (1991) 'Social Work, Modernity and Postmodernity', *Sociological Review*, 39 (4): 171–92.

McCartney, W. (1939) *Walls Have Mouths: a Record of Ten Years' Penal Servitude*, Left Book Club edn, London: Victor Gollancz.

McGuire, J. (ed.) (1995) *What Works: Reducing Reoffending*, Chichester: John Wiley.

McHale, B. (1992) *Constructing Postmodernism*, London: Routledge.

McWilliams, W. (1981) 'The Probation Officer at Court: from Friend to Acquaintance', *Howard Journal of Penology and Crime Prevention*, xx: 97–116.

—— (1983) 'The Mission to the English Police Courts 1876–1936' *Howard Journal of Penology and Crime Prevention*, xxii: 129–47.

—— (1985) 'The Mission Transformed: Professionalisation of Probation Between the Wars', *Howard Journal of Criminal Justice*, 24: 257–74.

Mair, G. (1991) 'What Works – Nothing or Everything?' *Home Office Research Bulletin*, 30: 3–8.

Marshall, T. H. (1946) 'Training for Social Work', in Nuffield College (ed.) *Training for Social Work*, London: Oxford University Press.

Martinson, R. (1974) 'What Works? Questions and Answers about Prison Reform', *The Public Interest*, 35: 22–54.

Matza, D. (1964) *Delinquency and Drift*, New York: Wiley.

Maxwell, R. (1956) *Borstal and Better: a Life Story*, London: Hollis & Carter.

May, T. (1991) *Probation: Politics, Policy and Practice*, Buckingham: Open University Press.

Means, R. and Smith, R. (1994) *Community Care: Policy and Practice*, London: Macmillan.

Mellor, A. and Dent, H. (1994) 'Preparation of the Child Witness for Court', *Child Abuse Review*, 13 (3): 165–76.

Merton, R. (1972) 'Insiders and Outsiders: a Chapter in the Sociology of Knowledge', in R. Merton *et al.* (eds), *Varieties of Political Expression in Sociology*, Chicago: University of Chicago Press.

Mestrovic, S. (1993) *The Barbarian Temperament: Toward a Postmodern Critical Theory*, London: Routledge.

Meyer, H., Borgatta, E. and Jones, W. (1963) *Girls at Vocational High: an Experiment in Social Work Intervention*, New York: Russell and Sage Foundation.

Moody, H. R. (1993) 'What is Critical Gerontology and Why is it Important?', in T. Cole, A. Achenbaum, P. Jackobi and R. Kastenbaum (eds) *Voices and Visions of Ageing: Toward a Critical Gerontology*, London: Springer Publishing Co. pp. xv–xii.

Morris, A., Giller, H., Szwed, E. and Geach, H. (1980) *Justice for Children*, London: Macmillan.

Mulhall, S. and Swift, A. (1992) *Liberals and Communitarians*, Oxford: Basil Blackwell.

Munday, B. (1972) 'What is Happening to Social Work Students?', *Social Work Today*, 3 (6).

NALGO (1989) *Social Work in Crisis*, London: NALGO.

National Audit Office (1989) *Home Office: Control and Management of Probation Services in England and Wales*, London: HMSO.

National Children's Home (1991) *Poverty and Nutrition Survey, 1991*, London: NCH.

Newman, J. and Clarke, J. (1994) 'Going about our Business? The Managerialization of Public Services', in J. Clarke, A. Cochrane and E. McLaughlin (eds) *Managing Social Policy*, London: Sage.

Newton, C. and Marsh, P. (1993) *Training in Partnership: Translating Interventions in Practice in Social Services*, York: Joseph Rowntree Foundation.

O'Connor, J. (1973) *The Fiscal Crisis of the State*, London: St James Press.

Oppenheim, C. (1993) *Poverty: the Facts*, London: Child Poverty Action Group.

Oppenheimer, M. (1975) 'The Unionisation of the Professions', *Social Policy*, 5 (5).

Otway, O. and Peake, A. (1994) 'Using a Facilitated Self-help Group for Women whose Children have been Sexually Abused', *Groupwork*, 7 (2): 153–62.

Owen, H. and Pritchard, J. (1993) *Good Practice in Child Protection*, London: Jessica Kingsley.

Page, M. (1992) *Crimefighters of London: a History of the Origins and Development of the London Probation Service 1876–1965*, London: Inner London Probation Service Benevolent and Educational Trust.

Page, R. and Baldock, J. (eds) (1994) *Social Policy Review*, 6, Canterbury: Social Policy Association.

Pardeck, J. T., Murphy, J. W. and Chung, W. S. (1994) 'Social Work and Postmodernism', *Social Work and Social Science Review*, 5 (2): 113–23.

Parker, R. (ed.) (1980) *Caring for Separated Children: Plans, Procedures and Priorities. A Report by a Working Party Established by the National Children's Bureau*, London: Macmillan.

Parry, N. and Parry, P. (1979) 'Social Work, Professionalism and the State', in N. Parry, M. Rustin and C. Satyamurti (eds), *Social Work, Welfare and the State*, London: Edward Arnold.

Parton, C. (1990) 'Women, Gender, Oppression and Child Abuse', in the Violence Against Children Study Group, *Taking Child Abuse Seriously: Contemporary Issues in Child Protection Theory and Practice*, London: Unwin Hyman.

Parton, C. and Parton, N. (1989a) 'Child Protection, the Law and Dangerousness', in O. Stevenson (ed). *Child Abuse: Public Policy and Professional Practice*, Hemel Hempstead: Harvester-Wheatsheaf.

—— (1989b) 'Women, the Family and Child Protection', *Critical Social Policy*, 24: 38–49.

Parton, N. (1985) *The Politics of Child Abuse*, London: Macmillan.

—— (1986) 'The Beckford Report: a Critical Appraisal', *British Journal of Social Work*, 16 (5): 511–30.

—— (1989) 'Child Abuse', in B. Kahan, (ed.) *Child Care Research, Policy and Practice*, London: Hodder & Stoughton.

—— (1990) 'Taking Child Abuse Seriously', in the Violence Against Children Study Group, *Taking Child Abuse Seriously: Contemporary Issues in Child Protection Theory and Practice*, London: Unwin Hyman.

—— (1991) *Governing the Family: Child Care, Child Protection and the State*, London: Macmillan.

—— (1994a) '"Problematics of Government", (Post)modernity and Social Work', *British Journal of Social Work*, 24 (1): 9–32.

—— (1994b) 'The Nature of Social Work under Conditions of (Post)modernity', *Social Work and Social Science Review*, 5, (2): 93–112.

Patel, P. (1990) 'Southall Boys', in Southall Black Sisters (ed.) *Against the Grain*: London.

Payne, M. (1992) 'Psychodynamic Theory within the Politics of Social Work Theory', *Journal of Social Work Practice*, 6 (2): 141–9.

Pearson, G. (1975) 'Making Good Social Workers: Bad Promises and Good Omens', in R. Bailey and M. Brake (eds), *Radical Social Work*, London: Edward Arnold.

Pearson, G., Treseder, J. and Yellolly, M. (eds) (1988) *Social Work and the Legacy of Freud*, Basingstoke: Macmillan.

Pease, K., Billingham, S. and Earnshaw, I. (1977) *Community Service Assessed in 1976*, Home Office Research Study No. 39, London: HMSO.

Pease, K., Durkin, P., Earnshaw, I., Payne, D. and Thorpe, J. (1975) *Community Service Orders*, Home Office Research Study No. 29. London: HMSO.

Peay, J. (1982) 'Dangerousness: Ascription or Description?', in P. Fieldman (ed.), *Developments in the Study of Criminal Behaviour*, vol. 2, *Violence*, Chichester: Wiley.

Percy-Smith, J. and Sanderson, I. (1992) *Understanding Local Needs*, London: Institute for Public Policy Research.

Perkin, H. (1969) *The Origins of Modern English Society 1790–1880*, London: Routledge & Kegan Paul.

Philips, A. (1993) *Democracy and Difference*, Cambridge: Polity Press.

Phillips, J. (1992a) *Private Residential Care: the Admission Process and Reactions of the Public Sector*, Aldershot: Avebury.

—— (1992b) 'The Future of Social Work with Older People', *Generations Review*, 2 (4).

Phillipson, C. (1994) 'Modernity, Post-modernity and the Sociology of Ageing: Reformulating Critical Gerontology', paper presented at XIIth World Congress of Sociology, Germany.

Phillipson, C. and Walker, A. (1986) *Ageing and Social Policy*, Aldershot: Gower.

Philp M. (1979) 'Notes on the Form of Knowledge in Social Work', *Sociological Review*, 27 (1): 83–111.

Phoenix, A. (1986) 'Theories of Gender and Black Families', in G. Weiner and M. Arnot (eds), *Gender under Scrutiny*, London: Unwin Hyman.

Pinch, S. (1994) 'Labour Flexibility and the Changing Welfare State: Is There a Post-Fordist Model?', in R. Burrows and B. Loader (eds), *Towards a Post-Fordist Welfare State*? London: Routledge.

Pinker, R. (1982) 'An Alternative View', in P. Barclay (Chair), *Social Workers: Their Roles and Tasks*, London: Bedford Square Press.

—— (1984) 'The Threat to Professional Standards in Social Work Education: a Response to Some Recent Proposals', *Issues in Social Work Education*, 4 (1): 5–15.

Pithers, D. (1989) 'A Guide through the Maze of Child Protection', *Social Work Today*, 20 (18): 18–19.

Pithouse, A. (1987) *Social Work: the Social Organisation of an Invisible Trade*, Aldershot: Gower Press.

Pollitt, C. (1990) *Managerialism and the Public Services*, Oxford: Basil Blackwell.

Pound, A. (1991) 'NEWPIN and child abuse', *Child Abuse Review*, 5: 7–10.

Power, M. (1994a) *The Audit Explosion*, London: Demos.

—— (1994b) 'The Audit Society', in A. G. Hopwood and P. Miller (eds), *Accounting as Social and Institutional Practice*, Cambridge: Cambridge University Press.

Powers, E. and Witmer, H. (1951) *An Experiment in the Prevention of Delinquency: the Cambridge-Somerville Youth Study*, New York: Columbia University Press.

Pozatek, E. (1994) 'The Problem of Certainty: Clinical Social Work in the Postmodern Era', *Social Work*, 39, (4): 396–403.

Preston-Shoot, M. and Agass, D. (1990) *Making Sense of Social Work: Psychodynamics, Systems and Practice*, London: Macmillan.

Pringle, R. and Watson, S. (1992) ''Women's Interests' and the Post-structuralist State', in M. Barrett and A. P. Phillips (eds), *Destabilizing Theory: Contemporary Feminist Debates*, Cambridge: Polity Press.

Prins, H. (1986) *Dangerous Behaviour, the Law and Mental Disorder*, London: Tavistock.

Radzinowicz, L. and Hood, R. (1981) 'A Dangerous Direction for Sentencing Reform', *Criminal Law Review*, pp. 776–61.

Rankin, G. (1970) 'Professional Social Work and the Campaign against Poverty', *Social Work Today*, 1 (10): 19–21.

Raynor, P. (1988) *Probation as an Alternative to Custody: a Case Study*, Aldershot: Avebury.

Raynor, P., Smith, D. and Vanstone, M. (1994) *Effective Probation Practice*, London: Macmillan.

Reakes, G. (1953) *The Juvenile Offender*, London: Christopher Johnson.

Reder, P., Duncan, S. and Gray, M. (1993) *Beyond Blame: Child Abuse Tragedies Revisited*, London: Routledge.

Reed Report (1992) *Review of Health and Social Services for Mentally Disordered Offenders and Others Requiring Similar Services*, London: Department of Health/Home Office.

Report of a Royal Society Study Group (1992) *Risk: Analysis, Perception and Management*, London: The Royal Society.

Rojek, C., Peacock, G. and Collins, S. (1988) *Social Work and Received Ideas*, London: Routledge.

Rose, N. (1985) *The Psychological Complex: Psychology, Politics and Society in England, 1869–1939*, London: Routledge & Kegan Paul.

—— (1993) 'Government, Authority and Expertise in Advanced Liberalism', *Economy and Society*, 22 (3): 283–99.

Rose, N. and Miller, P. (1992) 'Political Power Beyond the State: Problematics of Government', *British Journal of Sociology*, 43 (2): 173–205.

Rustin, M. (1989) 'The Politics of Post-Fordism: or the Trouble with 'New Times'', *New Left Review*, 175: 54–77.

—— (1994) 'Flexibility in Higher Education', in R. Burrows and B. Leader (eds) *Towards a Post-Fordist Welfare State?*, London: Routledge.

St John, J. (1961) *Probation – the Second Chance*, London: Vista Books.

Sands, R. G. and Nuccio, K. (1992) 'Postmodern Feminist Theory and Social Work', *Social Work*, 37 (6): 489–94.

Satyamurti, C. (1974) 'Women's Occupation and Social Change: the Case of Social Work', unpublished paper given to the 1974 British Sociological Association's Annual Conference.

Sayer, A. and Walker, D. (1992) *The New Social Economy*, Oxford: Blackwell.

Schorr, A. L. (1992) *The Personal Social Services: an Outsider's View*, York: Joseph Rowntree Foundation.

Scott, J. W. (1992) 'Deconstructing Equality-versus-Difference . . . or, the Uses of Post-structuralist Theory for Feminism', in L. McDowell and R. Pringle (eds) *Defining Women: Social Institutions and Gender Situations*, Cambridge: Polity Press in association with the Open University.

Secretary of State for Social Services (1974) *Report of the Inquiry into the Care and Supervision Provided in Relation to Maria Colwell*, London: HMSO.

—— (1988) *Report of the Inquiry into Child Abuse in Cleveland*, Cmnd 412, London: HMSO.

Seebohm Committee (1968) *Report of the Committee on Local Authority and Allied Personal Social Services*, Cmnd 3703, London: HMSO.

Seed, P. (1973) *The Expansion of Social Work in Great Britain*, London: Routledge & Kegan Paul.

Shilling, C. (1993) *The Body and Social Theory*, London: Sage.

Sibeon, R. (1991) 'A Contemporary Sociology of Social Work', in M. Davies (ed.), *The Sociology of Social Work*, London: Routledge.

Sibeon, R. (1992) 'Sociological Reflections on Welfare Politics and Social Work', *Social Work and Social Sciences Review*, 3 (3): 184–203.

Slater, J. (1967) *Approved School Boy*, London: William Kimber.

Smart, B. (1993) *Postmodernity*, London: Routledge.

Smith, E. D. (1957) 'Education and the Task of Making Social Work Professional', *Social Services Review*, 31, (March): 1–10.

Smith, M. (1965) *Professional Education for Social Work in Britain*, London: Allen & Unwin.

Social Services Committee (HC360) (1984) *Children in Care*, London: HMSO.

Social Services Inspectorate (1992) *Confronting Elder Abuse*, London: HMSO.

—— (1993) *Evaluating Performance in Child Protection: a Framework for the Inspection of Local Authority Social Services Practice and Systems*, London: HMSO.

Sone, K. (1994) 'The "At Risk" Trap', *Community Care* (10–16 Nov.): 16–17.

Squires, J. (ed.) (1993) *Principal Positions: Postmodernism and the Rediscovery of Value*, London: Lawrence & Wishart.

Stenson, K. (1993) 'Social Work Discourse and the Social Work Interview', *Economy and Society*, 22 (1): 42–76.

Stevenson, O. and Parsloe, P. (1993) *Community Care and Empowerment*, York: Joseph Rowntree Foundation.

Stewart, J. (1993a) 'Advance of the New Magistracy' *Local Government Management*, (Summer): 18–19.

—— (1993b) 'The Limitations of Government by Contract', *Public Money and Management* (July/Sept.): 7–12.

Stevenson, O. (1994) 'Social Work in the 1990s: Empowerment – Fact or Fiction?' in R. Page and J. Baldock (eds). *Social Policy Review*, 6, London: Social Policy Association, pp. 170–89.

Swanhunter, D. (1994) *Community Care in Practice*, London: Batsford.

Taylor, D. (1995) 'MP Backs Hols for Hooligans Shake-up', *Hull Daily Mail* (3 Jan.).

Taylor, G. (1993) 'Challenges from the Margins', in J. Clarke (ed.), *A Crisis in Care*, London: Sage.

Taylor, L., Lacey, R. and Bracken, D. (1980) *In Whose Best Interests?* London: Cobden Trust/MIND.

Taylor-Gooby, P. (1994) 'Postmodernism and Social Policy: a Great Leap Backwards?', *Journal of Social Policy*, 23 (3): 385–404.

Taylor-Gooby, P. and Lawson, R. (eds) (1993) *Markets and Managers: New Issues in the Delivery of Welfare*, Milton Keynes: Open University Press.

Titmuss, R. (1954) 'The Administrative Setting of Social Services', *Case Conference*, 1 (1): 3–8.

Todd, M. (1963) *The Probation Officer and his World*, London: Victor Gollancz.

—— (1964) *Ever Such a Nice Lady*, London: Victor Gollancz.

Tönnies, F. (1955) *Community and Association*, trans. C. Loomis, London: Routledge & Kegan Paul.

Twigg, J. and Atkin, K. (1994) *Carers Perceived: Policy and Practice in Informal Care*, Milton Keynes: Open Univerisity Press.

Ungerson, C. (1993) 'Payments for Caring – Mapping a Territory', in N. Deakin and R. Page (eds), *Paying For Welfare*, Aldershot: Avebury.

United Nations (1951) *Probation and Related Measures*, document E/CN.5/230, New York: United Nations.

—— (1954) *European Seminar on Probation, London 20–30 October 1952*, Document ST/TAA/SER.C/11, New York: United Nations.

Unsworth, C. (1987) *The Politics of Mental Health Legislation*, Oxford: Oxford University Press.

Wagner, P. (1994) *A Sociology of Modernity: Liberty and Discipline*, London: Routledge.

Walker, H. and Beaumont, B. (1981) *Probation Work: Critical Theory and Socialist Practice*, Oxford: Basil Blackwell.

Wardhaugh, J. and Wilding, P. (1993) 'Towards an Explanation of the Corruption of Care', *Critical Social Policy*, 37: 4–31.

Watson, J. (1939) *Meet the Prisoner*, London: Jonathan Cape.

—— (1969) *Which is the Justice?*, London: Allen & Unwin.

Wattam, C. (1992) *Making a Case in Child Protection*, London, NSPCC/Longman.

Webb, A. and Wistow, G. (1987) *Social Work, Social Care and Social Planning: the Personal Social Services since Seebohm*, London: Longman.

Webb, D. (1991) 'Puritans and Paradigms: a Speculation on the Form of New Moralities in Social Work', *Social Work and Social Sciences Review*, 2 (2): 146–59.

—— (1992) 'Competencies, Contracts and Cadres: Common Themes in the Social Control of Nurse and Social Work Education', *Journal of Interprofessional Care*, 6 (3): 223–30.

Wilkinson, R. G. (1994) *Unfair Shares: the Effects of Income Differences on the Welfare of the Young*, Ilford: Barnado's.

Williams, F. (1989) *Social Policy: a Critical Introduction*, Cambridge: Polity Press.

—— (1992) 'Somewhere Over the Rainbow: Universality and Diversity in Social Policy', in *Social Policy Review*, 4: 200–19.

—— (1993) 'Gender, Race and Class in British Welfare Policy', in A. Cochrane and J. Clarke (eds), *Comparing Welfare States*, London: Sage.

—— (1994) 'Social Relations, Welfare and the Post-Fordist Debate', in R. Burrows and B. Loader (eds), *Towards a Post-Fordist Welfare State*, London: Sage.

Wilson, D. (1974) 'Uneasy Bedfellows', *Social Work Today*, 5 (3): 9–12.

Wilson, R. (1949) 'Aims and Methods of a Department of Social Studies', *Social Work*, 6.

Wistow, G., Knapp, M., Hardy, B. and Allen, C. (1994) *Social Care in a Mixed Economy*, London: Open University Press.

Wood, D. (1988) 'Dangerous Offenders and the Morality of Protective Sentencing', *Criminal Law Review*, pp. 424–33.

Woodroofe, K. (1966) *From Charity to Social Work*, London: Routledge & Kegan Paul.

Woods, S. (1989) 'New Wave Management', *Work, Employment and Society*, 3 (3): 379–402.

Wootton, B. (1959) 'Daddy Knows Best', 166 (192): 248–61.

Wright Mills, C. (1970), *The Sociological Imagination*, Harmondsworth: Penguin.

Yeatman, A. (1994) *Postmodern Revisionings of the Political*, London: Routledge.

Yelloly, M. A. (1975) 'Professional Ideologies in British Social Work', unpublished PhD thesis, University of Leicester.

Young, J. (1971a) *The Drugtakers: the Social Meaning of Drug Use*, London: MacGibbon & Kee.

—— (1971b) 'The Role of the Police as Amplifiers of Deviancy, Negotiators of Reality and Translators of Fantasy: Some Consequences of Our Present System of Drug Control as Seen in Notting Hill', in S. Cohen (ed.), *Images of Deviance*, Harmondsworth: Penguin Books.

Younghusband, E. (1947) *Report on the Employment and Training of Social Workers*, Edinburgh: Constable.

—— (1951) *Report on the Employment and Training of Social Workers*, Edinburgh: T. A. Constable.

—— (1952) 'The Past and Future of Social Work', *Social Work*, 9 (4).

Zito Trust (1995) *Learning the Lessons*, London: Zito Trust.

Author index

Subject index